Practical Handbook of Veterinary Physiology

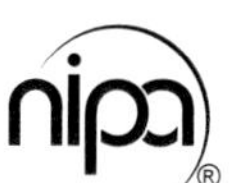

NIPA® GENX ELECTRONIC RESOURCES & SOLUTIONS P. LTD.
New Delhi-110 034

About the Author

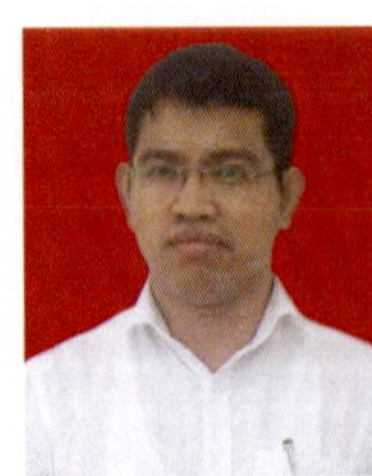

Dr. Bhabesh Mili graduated from the College of Veterinary Science, Assam Agricultural University, Khanapara, Assam, in 2010. He did his M.V.Sc. degree in Animal Physiology from the ICAR-National Dairy Research Institute, Karnal, Haryana, and Ph.D. degree in Veterinary Physiology from ICAR-Indian Veterinary Research Institute, Izanagar-243122, India. He has cleared ICAR-NET and ICAR-SRF. Dr. Mili has been working as an assistant professor at the College of Veterinary Sciences & Animal Husbandry, Jalukie, Peren district, Nagaland, under Central Agricultural University, Imphal, Manipur since 2016. He also worked as project scientist at the ICMR-Regional Medical Research Centre (NE Region), Dibrugarh-786001, Assam. Besides publishing popular articles and manuals, he has published two books, four book chapters, and 23 research papers in international and national peer-reviewed journals.

Practical Handbook of Veterinary Physiology A Comprehensive Guide to Undergraduate Students

Bhabesh Mili, M.V.Sc., Ph.D
Assistant Professor
Department of Veterinary Physiology and Biochemistry
College of Veterinary Sciences and Animal Husbandry
Central Agricultural University (Imphal)
Jalukie, Peren Dist., Nagaland-797110

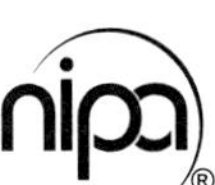

NIPA® GENX ELECTRONIC RESOURCES & SOLUTIONS P. LTD.
New Delhi-110 034

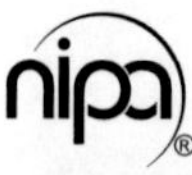

NIPA® GENX ELECTRONIC
RESOURCES & SOLUTIONS P. LTD.

101,103, Vikas Surya Plaza, CU Block
L.S.C. Market, Pitam Pura, New Delhi-110 034
Ph : +91 11 27341616, 27341717, 27341718
E-mail: newindiapublishingagency@gmail.com
Website: www.nipabooks.com
For customer assistance, please contact
Phone: + 91-11-27 34 17 17
Fax: + 91-11-27 34 16 16
E-Mail: feedbacks@nipabooks.com

ISBN: 978-81-19072-23-1

Composed and Designed by NIPA®.

Dedicated to My father
Mr. Someswar Mili
for his Everlasting Discipline, Moral and Ethical Values
My mother
Mrs. Iirawati Mili
for her Scarifies and Belief in Me and
My wife
Dr Haripriya Dutta
for her Enormous Patience, Support and Encouragement

Preface

Basic sciences like veterinary physiology, serve as the foundation upon which a veterinary graduate student builds his or her understanding of the veterinary sciences. The knowledge of veterinary physiology serves as a cornerstone for understanding pathophysiology, animal productivity, and treatment strategies.

Hence, an effort has been made to prepare a comprehensive handbook of veterinary physiology covering all practical's (experiments) to be conducted in hematology, cardiovascular system, digestive system, respiratory system, excretory system, endocrinology, physiology of reproduction, animal growth, environmental physiology & climatology, and animal behaviour, consulting different textbooks of veterinary physiology, research & review articles, as well as relevant websites, and the same has been acknowledged in the reference section.

All the analytical techniques have been written in a simplified language with brief importance, the normal physiological value of various parameters and interpretation for each experiment so that undergraduate students will have better insight into the subject. This handbook aims to serve the function of a manual as well as a practical textbook where all the pertinent experiments are compiled together for easy reference.

Being the first of its kind, any suggestions, ideas, and comments from the readers are highly appreciated for improvement in future editions.

3rd July, 2023 **Bhabesh Mili**

Contents

1

Applied Hematology

Bhabesh Mili and Amrit Gogoi

1.0. Introduction

Hematology is the study of blood and its constituents. Blood is a specialized fluid connective tissue, which consists of plasma (55-70%) and the formed elements (30-45%) that flow all over the body in the vessels of the cardiovascular system. Plasma comprises water (90-92%), proteins (6-7%), enzymes, hormones, lipids, and organic & inorganic constituents. The three major classes of plasma proteins include albumin, globulin, and fibrinogen. The organic elements include non-protein nitrogen (NPN) compounds (like urea, uric acid, creatine, creatinine, amino acids, glutathione, and xanthine), glucose, neutral fats, phospholipids, cholesterol and others. The inorganic constituents include calcium, phosphorus, magnesium, potassium, sodium, chlorine, sulfur, iodine, iron, copper, cobalt, manganese, zinc, selenium, and molybdenum; they contribute about 1 percent of the plasma.

Blood performs various functions by its constituents. The constituents of the blood are highly dynamic, and they inter shift from their reference values very quickly in any adverse condition. This is why; studies of blood cells and complete blood count (CBC) are important for accessing general health, diagnosing various diseases, and providing prognostic information when coupled with a thorough physical examination. The blood examination is performed routinely to diagnose hematological diseases, including certain hereditary diseases of the blood, and to determine the body's ability to respond to a hematological insult. The key parameters evaluated in the hemogram are ESR, PCV, Hb, TEC, MCV, MCHC, TLC, and DLC.

1.1. Collection of Blood Samples

The first step in the laboratory investigation of blood is to collect various types of specimens, whether whole blood, plasma, or serum. The choice of specimen depends upon the nature of investigations and the analytical procedure involved in the test. Blood samples are required to conduct various hematological, biochemical, microbiological, serological, or other tests, which can provide valuable diagnostic and prognostic information. The number of tests and type of study will decide how much blood is required. Normally, about 8-10% of total blood volume can be collected at a time safely, if required. Blood should be collected and preserved with appropriate anticoagulants for hematological tests.

Materials required

- Needles, syringes, scissors, cotton, absolute alcohol, blood collection vials and tourniquet.

Procedure

- Small amounts of blood can be collected by pricking the ear tip under aseptic conditions in order to perform different instant tests such as blood grouping, bleeding time, clotting time, etc.

For large quantities, collect the blood sample by venipuncture as follows:

- Collect the blood sample from a suitable vein with an appropriate hypodermic needle size. The site of blood collection and needle size differ between species (Table 1.1) in animals.
- Locate the vein from where the blood is to be drawn.
- Clip the hair and use absolute alcohol or sprit to sterilize the area.
- Raise the vein either by using a tourniquet or by applying pressure with your fingers.
- Connect a well sharpened sterile needle into a syringe, and then insert the needle into the raised vein. After inserting the needle into the vein, gently withdraw the syringe plunger or piston. If blood appears to be flowing from the needle, withdraw the required amount of blood directly into the syringe. Don't force the piston to pull blood. Because it has the potential to cause hemolysis.
- After collecting blood, apply a sterile swab with gentle pressure over the punctured site and withdraw the needle.

Table 1.1: Site and appropriate size of hypodermic needle for blood collection from animals:

Species	Site	Needle gauge
Cattle, Buffalo & Horse	Jugular vein	16 – 18
Sheep & Goat	Jugular vein	18 – 20
Pig	Anterior vena cava & ear vein	20 - 22
Dog	Recurrent tarsal vein & saphenous vein	20 – 22
Cat	Recurrent tarsal vein & saphenous vein	20 – 25
Rabbit	Cardiac puncture and marginal ear vein	18 – 20
Rat & Mouse	Cardiac puncture and cutting of tail	22 – 25
Bird	Wing vein	20 - 25

Handling of Blood Sample

After blood collection, the vial should be gently closed, and then the blood should be mixed with an anticoagulant by repeated inversion or circular movements of the vial. Rough handling or severe shaking may lead to hemolysis, which will lead to erroneous results.

Precautions

Animals should be allowed to calm down before the collection of blood to avoid stress- related changes on the hemogram. Avoid collecting blood from the arteries since it is painful and can cause damage and necrosis to the arterial vessels. The hypodermic needle and syringe must be properly sterilized and dried before blood collection. Water or any hypotonic moisture may rupture the RBCs (hemolysis). Use a standard needle gauge for blood collection from a particular species. The needle of gauges has various drawbacks, such as a decrease in blood flow rate, velocity, turbulence, and hemolysis. The needle should be separated from the syringe after the collection of blood and transferred slowly to the blood collection vial. Platelet counts should be performed within 4 hours of the blood samples being collected.

1.2. Anticoagulants

Anticoagulants are inorganic substances that prevent blood from clotting and hence keep it in a liquid state. *In-vitro* blood is physiologically liquid, but when it is drawn outside from the blood vessel, it clots within minutes. The Table 1.2 below shows the most common anticoagulants used for the collection of blood samples for routine hematological procedures.

Table 1.2: List of anticoagulants and their mechanism of action:

Anticoagulants	Quantity required	Advantages	Disadvantages	Mechanism of action
1. Heparin	0.2 mg/mL (20 IU) of blood.	Use for routine hematological procedures, blood gas determination and pH assays.This anticoagulant is best for the osmotic fragility test.	An excess amount causes shrinkage of cells and inhibits platelet interaction.Heparin is not recommendedfor study of the morphology of cells because of poor staining properties of WBC.	Conversion of prothrombin to thrombin & prevent action of thrombin on fibrinogen.
2. EDTA (Ethylenediamine tetraacetic acid)	1.0 mg/mL of blood.	Suitable for routine blood studies. EDTA is the preferred anticoagulant for studies of blood morphology, quantitative methods involving cells and erythrocyte indices. It is also suitable for totalprotein and BUN estimation.	Excess amounts cause shrinkage of RBCs, resultingin errors in PCV, MCV, and MCHC. This anticoagulant is not useful for blood transfusion, estimation of calcium, magnesium, sodium, potassium, etc.	Precipitate calcium as salt (strong chelating agents).
3. Oxalates: a) Potassium oxalates b) Ammonium oxalates	4.0 mg of (a) and 6.0 mg of (b) should be mixed for 8-10 mL of blood.	Suitable for routine blood studies.	Not suitable for blood transfusion, NPN and BUN.	Unites with Ca^{++} to form insoluble calcium oxalate.
4. Sodium citrate (3.8% solution)	2.5 mL/10 mL of bloodsolution to be dried in sample test tube.	Mainly used in blood transfusions. Sodium citrate is the anticoagulant of choice for studies of coagulation. It is also used for the estimation of ESR in a 4:1 ratio (4 volumes of blood are added to 1 volumes of sodium citrate) by Westergren method.		Precipitate calcium as salt.
5. Sodium Fluoride	10.0 mg of (a) and 1.0 mg of (b) should be mixed for 1.0 mL of blood.	Suitable for blood glucoseestimation.	It can't be used in other estimation.	Precipitate calcium as salt. Inhibits enzyme enolase.

1.3. Separation of Blood Constituents

The blood tends to clot after it is withdrawn from the blood vessel. After the removal of the clot, the leftover fluid is known as serum. Hence, the serum is blood plasma devoid of fibrinogen and other clotting factors. Plasma is the liquid component of blood. If blood is treated with an anticoagulant immediately after being drawn outside the blood vessel, the liquid state of the blood is maintained. If such a blood sample is spun, the liquid fraction separates from the cells and is referred to as plasma.

Plasma – Fibrinogen=Serum

Defibrinated blood is a mixture of blood cells and serum, which is obtained after the removal of fibrin clots from the blood.

Materials required

- Fresh blood, anticoagulant, vials or tubes, conical flask, glass rod or bead, centrifuge tube, centrifugation machine, cryovial, etc.

Procedure for separation of plasma

- Collect the blood sample in anticoagulant-containing vials or tubes.
- Gently mix the vial containing the anticoagulated blood sample.
- After mixing, centrifuge the vial at 3000 rpm for 15-20 minutes. This will give three layers: from top to bottom- plasma, buffy coat (leucocytes and platelets) and erythrocytes.
- Carefully transfer the supernatant fluid (plasma) into a cryovial for future use. Take cautious not to disturb or transfer any cells from the cell layer.

Procedure for separation of serum

- Collect the blood sample and then transfer it in a tube with no anticoagulant.
- Allow the tube to clot for 30-45 minutes in a slanting position at room temperature. This will aid in the clotting of the blood.
- After clotting, centrifuge the vial at 3000 rpm for 20 minutes.
- The supernatant fluid part is the serum, which should be transferred carefully into a cryovial or storage vial for further use. Take cautious not to disturb or transfer any cells. The normal serum is clear and light yellow in colour.

Defibrination procedure

- Take 25 mL of a freshly drawn blood sample and place it in a 125 mL Erlenmeyer flask containing 3.4 mm glass beads.
- Rotate the flask for about 5-10 minutes or until the beads are covered with fibrin.
- Remove the fibrin clot; the remaining fluid is the defibrinated blood.

Preservation of Blood Constituents

Plasma, serum, and defibrinated blood samples can be preserved at refrigerated temperatures for different time periods. The Table 1.3 below shows the appropriate temperatures routinely employed for the preservation of plasma, serum, and defibrinated blood samples.

Table 1.3: Ideal temperature for preservation of plasma, serum, and defibrinated blood:

Sample type	Temperature	Duration
Plasma	4°C -20°C	24 hours Up to 6 months
Serum	4°C -20°C	24 hours Up to 1 your
Defibrinated blood	4°C -20°C	24 hours Up to 1 month

1.4. Bleeding Time and Clotting Time

Bleeding time (BT) is the time taken from a small, standardized wound to a complete cessation of bleeding. Bleeding from the blood capillaries ceases after the formation of platelet plugs at the cut ends of the capillaries. This process is called hemostasis. First, there is the formation of temporary soft platelet plugs (primary plugs) at the injury site. Then, an insoluble fibrin clot (secondary plugs) seals the cut or injured vessels and stops the bleeding, which is known as coagulation. Bleeding time depends on the function of the platelets and the integrity of the blood vessels. This test is performed before any surgical procedure or if there is a history of bleeding.

1.4.a. Determination of Bleeding Time (Duke's Method)

- Sterile razor or shaving blade, cotton swabs, sterilized needle, filter paper, etc.

Regents

- Alcohol (70%) or sprit.

Procedure

- The skin of the ear, nose, foot pad, and inside of the lip are generally preferred sites to determine bleeding time.
- After site selection, shave the area as needed with a sterile razor or shaving blade; if necessary, sterilize the area with 70% alcohol or rectified spirit.
- After complete drying, puncture a moderately deep (3-4 mm deep) hole and record the time.
- Let the blood flow freely without squeezing or applying any pressure. Go on wiping the blood at 15-second intervals until the bleeding stops.
- Record the time when the bleeding stopped completely.
- Then count the number of spots on the filter paper and express the result in minutes.
- Calculate the bleeding time using the formula below. The result may be obtained by dividing the difference between the initial time and the cessation of bleeding.

BT= No. of drops of blood on the filter paper x15 seconds or BT= Time at cessation of bleeding (T_2) -Time at puncture (T_1)

1.4.b. Clotting Time

Clotting time can be estimated by two methods:

1. Slide method
2. Capillary glass tube method

1.4.b.1. Slide method

- Glass slide, stopwatch, cotton and sterilized lancet.

Reagents

- Sprit or 70% alcohol.

Procedure

- Sterilize the area to be pricked.
- Prick the tip of the ear to allow blood to flow freely. Start the stopwatch (initial time).

- Put two or three drops of blood on the glass slide.
- At every 15 second interval, a needle is drawn through the drops of blood until it picks up a fibrin thread.
- Pause the stopwatch when a fibrin thread is hanging from the needle. Take note of the time (final time).

1.4.b.2. Capillary Glass Tube Method

- Capillary tube (1 mm diameter), stopwatch, cotton and sterilized lancet.

Reagents

- Sprit or 70 % alcohol.

Procedure

- Puncture the chosen bleeding site according to the procedure described in the determination of bleeding time. Then, without pressing, let the blood to flow freely.
- Draw a large drop of blood into the capillary tube by dipping one of its end into the drop in an oblique way. Approximately 3/4th of the tube should be filled.
- Take note the time (the initial time). After 2 minutes, break off a small portion of the capillary tube very carefully at 30-second intervals.
- Breaking should be continued until there is a hanging of a broken fragment of the tube with a fine thread of the clot. Take note of the time (final time). The time it takes for blood to clot is measured in minutes.

Clotting time=Final time – Initial time

Blood clotting time

Normal blood clotting time differs from species to species (Table 1.4). Most marine mammals and reptiles have delayed *in vitro* blood clotting times, which appears to be due to a lack of blood clotting factor XII or Hageman factor. However, avian blood clots are extremely rapid.

Table 1.4: Reference intervals for blood clotting time in domestic animals:

Parameters	Units	Dog	Cat	Cattle	Horse	Pig	Sheep	Goat
Clotting time	Time (minutes)	3.0 –13.0	4.5 –8.0	3.0 - 15.0	4.0 –15.0	2.5– 4.0	1.0-6.0	3.0 – 12.0

Prolong bleeding time and clotting time

- Thrombocytopenia due to aplastic anemia, idiopathic thrombocytopenic purpura (ITP), drug such as non-steroidal anti-inflammatory drugs (NASIDs), etc
- Liver diseases, deficiency of vitamin C, vitamin K, etc.
- Hereditary causes such as haemophilia A (called factor VIII deficiency), haemophilia B, prekallikrein, von Willebrand disease (vWD), etc.

1.5. Erythrocyte Sedimentation Rate

Blood in the circulatory system is always in motion. When blood with an anticoagulant is allowed to stand in a narrow vertical tube *in vitro*, the cells settle down gradually due to a higher specific gravity than plasma. The rate at which erythrocytes (red blood cells) settle down for a certain period is known as the "Erythrocyte Sedimentation Rate" (ESR) and is measured in mm. ESR can be determined by two methods.

a) Wintrobe method

b) Westergren method

1.5.a. Wintrobe Method

- Anticoagulant added blood sample, dry syringe with 4-6 inch long needle (16- 18 gauze), wintrobe tube and wintrobe stand. The wintrobe tube is 12 cm long with a bore diameter of 2 mm. It is calibrated from 0-100 mm from above downwards for ESR and 0-100 mm from below upwards for haematocrit.

Procedure

- Fill the Wintrobe tube with anticoagulant-added blood sample to the mark "0" with a Pasteur pipette.
- Allow them to stand vertically and completely undisturbed condition in the Wintrobe stand.
- Take note of the reading after an hour.

1.5.b. Westergren Method

Materials required

- Westergren tube: It is a straight pipette or tube that is 30 cm long and 2.5 mm in internal diameter. It is calibrated from 0 to 200 mm.

- Westergren stand or rack: It is to accommodate Westergren tubes in a vertical position. It can accommodate six Westergren tubes at a time.
- Syringe and needle (2 mL volume).
- 3.8% Sodium citrate (Dissolve 38.0 g of sodium citrate in 1.0 liter of distilled water in a sterile glass bottle).
- Spirit and cotton swabs.

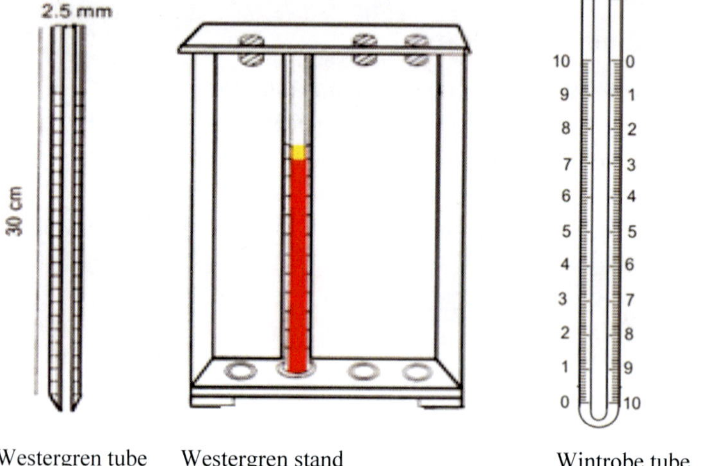

Westergren tube Westergren stand Wintrobe tube

Fig. 1.1: Estimation of ESR using Wintrobe tube and Westergren tube.

Procedure

- Fill the Westergren tube with the anticoagulant-added blood sample up to the "0" marks.
- Then place the tube upright in a Westergren stand.
- Allow the tube to stand in an undisturbed condition.
- Take note of the reading after an hour.

Reference value of ESR in domestic animals

In animals, normal ESR varies greatly from species to species. The ESR is affected by age, pregnancy, sex, and other factors. The reference interval for ESR in various domestic animals is shown in Table 1.5 below.

Table 1.5: Reference intervals for ESR in domestic animals:

Species	ESR
Cattle	2.4 mm per 7 hour
Horse	2-12 mm per 10 minutes
Pig	1-14 mm per hour
Sheep	0-1 mm per hour
Goat	0-1 mm per hour
Dog	6-10 per hour
Chicken	2-4mm per 7 hour

Increased ESR

- Physiological conditions -Pregnancy, exercise, old age, etc.
- Pathological conditions- Acute & chronic infections, anemia of all types, collagen disorders, malignancy, autoimmune disorders (Such as rheumatoid artrities and lupus), hypothyroidism, etc.
- Rapid ESR is observed in newborn piglets when the sow's diet does not contain enough iron.

Decreased ESR

- Physiological conditions- High altitude polycythemia (physiological polycythemia).
- Pathological conditions- Polycythemia, afibrinogenaemia, sickle cell anemia, hereditary spherocytosis, etc.

1.6. Estimation of Haemoglobin

Haemoglobin (Hb) is a complex iron-containing conjugated protein and is composed of haem and globin. Hb has a molecular weight of 66,000 to 69,000. Haem is responsible for haemoglobin's red colour. Biosynthesis of haemoglobin is a complex process and is started in the rubricyte or polychrmatophil erythroblast stage of red blood cell genesis (erythropoiesis). Hb has four polypeptide chains- alpha, beta, gamma and delta. Hbs are classified into two main types based on their physiological functions: adult (HbA) and fetal (HbF) haemoglobins. HbA is composed of two alpha and two beta polypeptide chains. In contrast to HbA, fetal Hb has two alpha and two gamma polypeptide chains.

The primary function of Hb is to transport O_2 from the lungs to the tissue and CO_2 from the tissue to the lungs. Hb also serves as an excellent body buffer system. The levels of Hb directly reflect the ability of the erythron to transport O_2.

There are many methods to estimate the Hb concentration of blood. The following are the most commonly used methods:

a) Sahli's acid haematin method

b) Cyanmethemoglobin method

1.6.a. Sahli's acid Haematin Method

Sahli's acid haematin method is the simplest and cheapest method for the estimation of Hb concentration in blood. Diluted acid (N/10 HCI) converts the Hb of the erythrocytes into acid haematin. The resulting stable brown colour of acid haematin is matched with standard glass filters or rods, which provide a reading in g/dL of blood as well as a percentage. The intensity of the stable brown colour of the solution depends upon the acid haematin.

Materials required

Sahli's (sahli - Adams) Haemoglobinometer consist (Fig.1.2) of:

(i) Haemoglobin pipette: It is a straight capillary pipette calibrated with 20.0 μL for drawing blood.

(ii) Haemoglobin tube: It is a round tube calibrated in g/dL on one face and on the other face in percentage (%).

(iii) Comparator box: It is a rectangular box that provides accommodation for the haemoglobin tube in the middle and a non-fading standard brown glass filter on either side for matching the colour.

(iv) A glass stirrer's rod.

(v) A dropper and Pasteur pipette.

(vi) A vial for N/10 hydrochloric acid (HCI).

Reagents and sample

- N/10 HCI, distilled water and anticoagulant mixed whole blood.

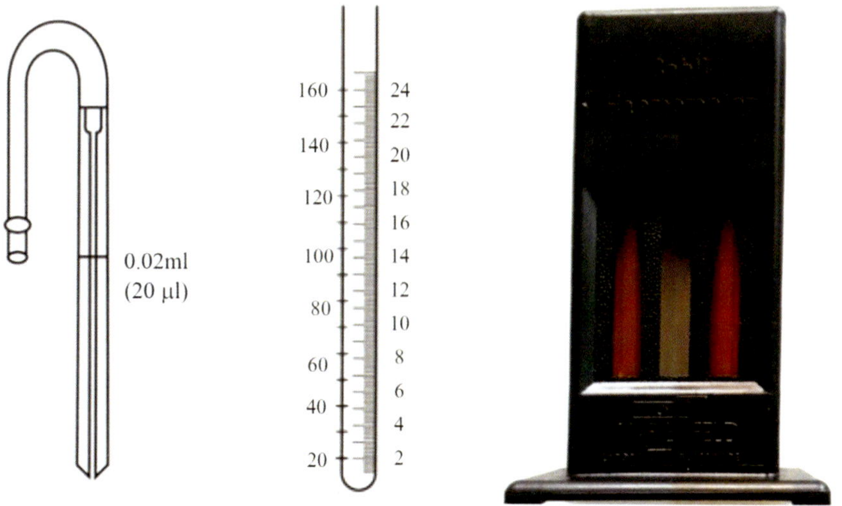

Haemoglobin pipette Haemoglobin tube Comparator box with a brown glass standard

Fig. 1.2: Haemeglobinometer for estimation of Hb concentration in blood.

Procedure

- Clean and dry all of the haemoglobinometer's glass components.
- Take N/10 HCI up to 2 marks in the haemoglobin tube.
- Draw the mixed blood up to 20 μL in a haemoglobin pipette. Wipe the tip and carefully discharge the blood into the haemoglobin tube containing N/10 HCI.
- Shake the tube well and leave it for at least 2-3 minutes to allow the acid haematin complex to develop.
- Put it in the visual comparator box. Then, drop by drop, dilute the brown-coloured acid haematin solution with distilled water, thoroughly mix it with the stirrer after each drop of distilled water, and compare the colour to the glass standard.
- The stirrer should be taken out during matching. Hold the instrument between your eye and the light while matching the colour every time. When the colour of the haemoglobin tube matches the colour of the comparator, remove it from the comparator.
- Take note of the g/dL calibration from the haemoglobin tube at the level of the lower meniscus. Hb levels in blood are measured in g per 100 nL of blood, or g%.

1.6.b. Cyanmethemoglobin Method

Hb is converted into a red-colored complex cyanmathemoglobin in the presence of potassium cyanide and ferricyanide at alkaline pH, which is detected using a photoelectric colorimeter at 540 nm wavelength. The colour intensity is proportional to the Hb content in the blood.

Materials required

- Spectrophotometer or photoelectric colorimeter, test tube, pipette, blood, etc.

Reagents

- Drabkin's solution, cyanmethemoglobin standard solution with a known haemoglobin value and anticoagulant-mixed blood sample. The composition of drabkin's solution is as follows:

Sodium bicarbonate	1.0g
Potassium cyanide	0.05g
Potassium ferricyanide	0.20g
Distilled water up to	1000 mL

Procedure

- Take three test tubes and mark them as 'T' (unknown or test sample), 'S' (standard), and 'B' (blank).
- Pipette blood, drabkin's solution, cyanmethemoglobin standard solution, and distilled water into all marked test tubes as follows:

	Blank	**Standard**	**Test**
Drabkin's solurion	5 mL	-	5 mL
Cyanmethemoglobin standard	-	5 mL	-
Blood	-	-	20 uL

- Mix the contents of the above tubes well and allow them to stand at room temperature for 5 minutes.
- Read the Optical Density (OD) of the test and standard against Drabkin's solution (blank) at 540 nm wavelengths on a colorimeter or spectrophotometer.
- Calculate the Hb% in the blood sample using the formula below.

  Hb in g% = (OD Test / OD Standard) x cone of standard in mg% x 0.251

  = (OD Test / OD Standard) x 60 X 0.251

  = (OD Test / OD Standard) x 15.06

Reference value of Hb concentration

Hb concentrations in the blood vary greatly among species (Table 1.6) in animals. It is also influenced by age, sex, muscular activity, season, excitement, etc.

Table 1.6: Reference intervals for Hb concentration in domestic animals:

Species	Cattle	Goat	Sheep	Pig	Horse	Dog	Cat	Chicken
Hemoglobin (gm/dL)	8-15	8-12	9-15	10-16	11.5-16	12-18	10-15	6.8-11.3

Increased Hb concentration

- Physiological conditions- Newborn, high altitude, exercise, excessive sweating, hemoconcentration due to severe vomiting, diarrhoea, etc.
- Pathological conditions -Polycythemia vera, chronic kidney diseases, lung diseases like emphysema, chronic carbon monoxide poison, etc.

Decreased Hb concentration

- Physiological condition -Hemodilution e.g., pregnancy.
- Pathological conditions- Anemia, ADH secreting pituitary tumour, hemoglobinopathies such as thalassemia, sickle cell anemia, etc.

1.7. Packed Cell Volume or Haematocrit

In general, blood corpuscle volumes are lower than plasma volumes. The ratio of corpuscles to plasma is expressed as the haematocrit value. The Greek word 'crit' means separate, so hematocrit refers to the separation of plasma from whole blood. The whole blood can be separated into three compartments by centrifugation: (i) the erythrocyte mass at the bottom, (ii) a white to grey layer of leucocytes and thrombocytes above the erythrocyte mass known as the Buffy coat, and (iii) the blood plasma. The masses of the three layers are separated gradually based on their specific gravity. Packed cell volume (PCV) is thus the proportion of total volume occupied by packed erythrocytes when a certain volume of anticoagulant-mixed blood is centrifuged at a specific rate. It provides a rapid hemogram and a rough estimation of total leucocytes by measuring the thickness of the Buffy coat.

Methods for the estimation of PCV

PCV can be determined by two methods:

a) Wintrobe method (Macro-hematocrit method)

b) Microhematocrit method (Micro-method)

1.7.a. Wintrobe Method

Materials required

1. The wintrobe hematocrit tube is 11 cm long and has an interior diameter of 3 mm. The volume is equivalent to about 1 mL of whole blood.
2. Hematocrit frame.
3. Centrifuge machine, and Pasteur pipette with a narrow delivery tip.

Reagents and sample

- Fresh whole blood and anticoagulant.

Procedure

- Gently mix the vial containing the anticoagulated blood sample.
- Fill the blood into the hematocrit tube up to mark 10 with a Pasteur pipette.
- The tip of the pipette should always remain below the advancing level of blood to avoid the formation of bubbles.
- Then, centrifuge the blood at 3000 rpm for 30 minutes. After completion, place the tube in a hematocrit frame.
- Take note of the volume on the right side of the scale. The result should be expressed as a percentage (%).

$$\text{PCV or hematocrit } (\%) \ \frac{\text{Height of the packed erythrocytes in mm}}{\text{Total height of the column in mm}} \times 100$$

1.7.b. Microhematocrit Method

The microhematocrit method has an advantage over the Wintrobe method because it requires less blood, takes less time, traps less plasma and is more accuracy. However, this method has limitations. It necessitates specific reading equipment as well as an unclear buffy coat.

Materials required

1. Microhematocrit centrifuge.
2. Capillary tubes (75 mm x 1.0 mm) - Heparinized capillary tubes have to be used when the blood sample does not contain an anticoagulant. Plain capillary tubes can be used for anticoagulant- mixed blood samples.

Reagents and sample

- Fresh blood and anticoagulant.

Procedure

- Gently mix the vial containing the anticoagulated blood sample.
- Put one end of the capillary tube on the blood's surface. Capillary action causes blood to enter the capillary tube. Remove the capillary tube when it is 3/4th full and seal one end with wax.
- Place the capillary tube into the slot of the hematocrit centrifuge with the sealed end towards the outside, and balance it against another tube of the same size on the opposite side of the centrifuge head.
- Then centrifuge at 10,000 rpm for 5 minutes. The PCV is read using a specific reading instrument after centrifugation.

Reference value of PCV (%)

The reference value of PCV % varies greatly among species (Table 1.7) in animals.

Table 1.7: Reference intervals for PCV (%) in domestic animals:

Species	Cattle	Goat	Sheep	Pig	Horse	Dog	Cat	Chicken
PCV (%)	24-46	22-38	27-45	32-50	34-45	37-55	30-45	27-42

In Wintrobe hematocrit, if the buffy coat is 1 mm or less, then 0.4 mm is equivalent to 1000 leucocytes. Above 1 mm is equivalent to 2000 leucocytes, however with leucopenia, there may be no Buffy coat.

Increased PCV

- Haemoconcentration.
- Polycythaemia.

Decreased PCV

- Bone marrow depression.
- Anemia.

1.8. Total Erythrocyte Count

Erythrocytes are anucleated, biconcave, elongated to spherical, non-motile cells that circulate in the blood of mammals. However, erythrocytes in birds are elliptical and have nuclei. Erythrocytes serve a variety of functions, but their main function is the transportation of respiratory gas. The life- span of erythrocytes in several domestic animals are: dog: 110 to 130 days (118 days); cat: 70-80 days; horse: 140-150 days; adult cattle, sheep, & goats: 125-150 days; lambs & calves: 50-100 days; chicken: 20-30 days; and ducks: 0-40 days.

Total erythrocyte count (TEC) provides information about erythropoiesis, polycythemia (an increase in the number of erythrocytes or RBCs above the reference value for TEC), oligocythemia (a decrease in the number of RBCs below reference value) and whether the subject is suffering from an anemic condition or not.

Materials required

(i) Compound microscope.

(ii) Haemocytometer consisting of:

a. Neubauer's counting chamber: The thick glass slide is divided into three platforms, two lateral ones and one center, by trenches. The central platform is divided into two halves with the help of a trench, giving it an 'H'-shaped appearance. The central platform is 1/10 mm lower than the platforms on either side. The central platform has two counting chambers named Neubauer's counting chamber for counting RBCs and WBCs. Each Neubauer's counting chamber consists of nine (9) sq. mm (3 mm X 3 mm). This area is divided by triple lines into nine (9) large equal squares, each having an area of 1 sq mm (1 mm X 1 mm). Of these, the four large squares at the corners are used for the enumeration of WBCs, while the large square in the center is used for the enumeration of erythrocytes. The large central square is further divided into 25 medium squares. Each medium square is further divided into 16 small squares, each having an area of 1/16 mm.

b. Coverslip.

c. RBC diluting pipette: The RBC diluting pipette has two markings on it: 0.5 at the bottom, and 101 at the top.

(iii) Sterile needle for puncturing the ear and sterile cotton.

Reagents and sample

- Blood sample and RBC diluting fluids.

The most common RBC diluting fluids are as follows:

1. Hayem's fluid: It contains

a) Mercuric chloride 0.25g: It acts as a preservative, anti-fungal, and antibacterial agent.

b) Sodium sulphate 2.50g: It acts as an anticoagulant and prevents rouleaux formation.

c) Sodium chloride 0.50g: It maintains isotonicity so that RBCs remain suspended in the fluid.

d) Distilled water up to 100.00 mL.

2. Toisson's fluid: It contains

a) Sodium sulphate 4.00 g

b) Sodium chloride 0.50 g

c) Glycerin 15.00 mL

d) Distilled water add upto100.00 mL

3. Gower's fluid: It contains

a) Sodium sulphate 12.50 g

b) Glacial acetic acid: 33.3 mL

c) Distilled water 200.00 mL

4. Formal citrate solution: It contains

a) Trisodium citrate 3.00 g

b) Formalin (conc.) 1.0 mL

c) Distilled water add upto 100.00 mL

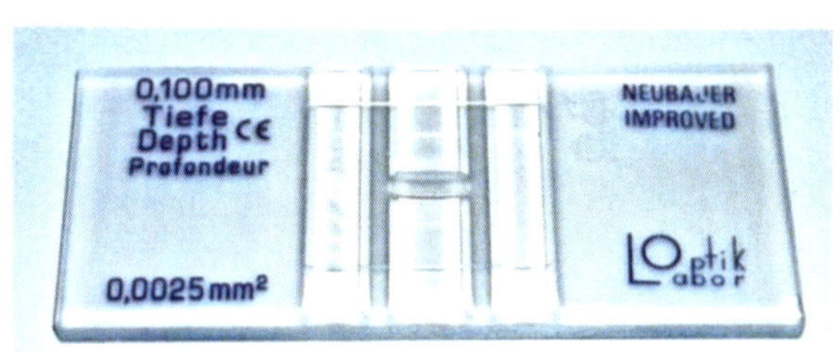

Haemocytometer

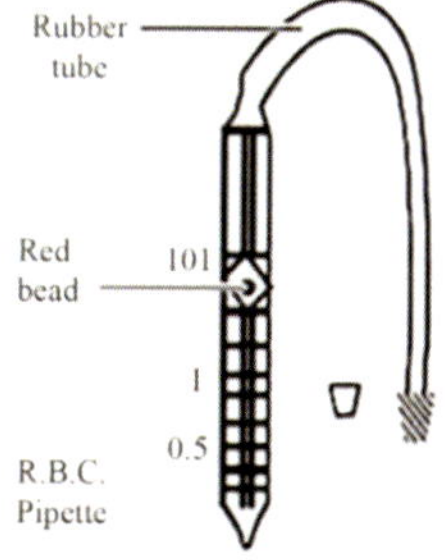

RBC diluting pipette

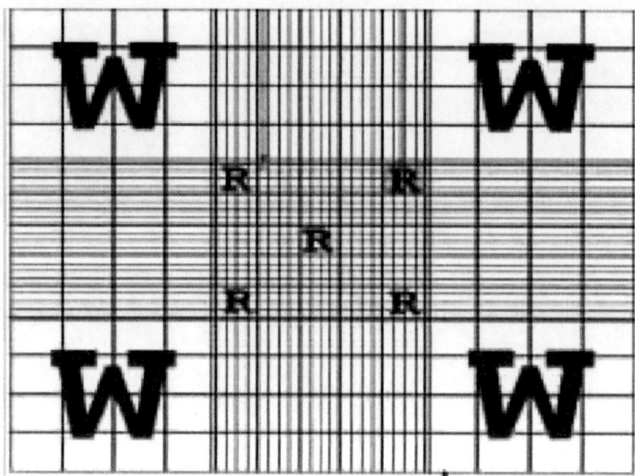

View of Neubauer's counting chamber under microscope

Fig.1.3: Haemocytometer and RBC diluting pipette for estimation of TLC.

Procedure

- Place the coverslip over the central platform of the haemocytometer. The ridges on both sides of the centre platform support the coverslip.
- Mount the slide on the mechanical stage of the microscope and focus the Neubauer's counting chamber under a low-power (10x) objective.
- Gently mix the vial containing the anticoagulated blood sample. Draw the blood up to 0.5 calibrated marks in the RBC diluting pipette. If blood is drawn beyond the mark, the excess blood should be removed by stroking the tip of the pipette with the tip of the finger. Then, the tip of the pipette should be wiped with cotton.
- Dip the tip of the pipette in the diluting fluid and suck the diluting fluid up to the upper mark above the bulb (101 in case of RBC) for dilution of blood. This gives a dilution of 1 into 200.
- Mix the blood with diluting fluid for about 3-5 minutes by rotating it in your palm, keeping the pipette always horizontal.
- Put the coverslip on the central platform of Neubauer's counting chamber, place it on the microscope stage, and focus it again.
- Discard 2-3 drops of diluting fluid from the pipette after proper mixing.
- Wipe the tip of the RBC diluting pipette, then charge (one drop) the diluted blood at the edge of the coverslip at an angle of 30° to the horizontal.

- Avoid any air bubbles. Do not allow blood to flow over the coverslip as it will give a false count.
- Allow the diluted blood to flow under the coverslip to settle the cells.
- Finally, focus Neubauer's counting chamber on the high-power (40x) objective.
- Move the chamber to the upper left corner block of 16 small (tertiary) squares and adjust the illumination.
- Count the erythrocytes in four corner squares (two uppers and two lowers) and one central square.
- The cells that touched the left and upper border lines of the square can be considered for those squares, ignoring those that are falling on the right and lower border.

Calculation

1.	One primary square has 1 mm length, 1 mm width	
2.	The primary square is divided into 5 X 5	= 25 secondary squares
3.	So, the surface area of one secondary square will be (Length X Width)	$= \frac{1}{5} \times \frac{1}{5} = \frac{1}{25}$ mm^2
4.	The cubic volume of one secondary square will be (surface area X height) So, the cubic volume of five secondary squares will be	$\frac{1}{25} = mm^2 X \frac{1}{10} mm$ $\frac{1}{250} = mm^3$ $\frac{1}{250} = 5 X mm^3$ $\frac{1}{50} = mm^3$
5.	If the blood is taken up to the 0.5 mark in the RBC pipette, then the dilution factor will be	= 200
6.	Let us assume the total number of cells counted in the 5 secondary squares (80 small squares) is "X" in mm^3 of blood	
7.	Therefore, the number of erythrocytes present in 1 mm^3 of diluted blood will be	$= 50 \times X$
8.	Now, it can be said that $50 \times X$ number of erythrocytes are present in 1 mm^3 volume of undiluted blood	
9.	Here, as blood is diluted and the dilution factor is 200,so the number of RBCs in the examined diluted blood is	$= 50 \times X \times 200/mm^3$ $=X \times 10^4/mm^3$

It is generally expressed as______million/ mm^3 or_______$\times$ 10 mm^3

Reference value forTEC

The reference value for erythrocyte counts varies greatly among species (Table 1.8) in animals. TEC also varies according to factors like age, sex, exercise, nutritional status, lactation, pregnancy, egg production, excitement, blood volume, stage of the estrus cycle, breed, environmental temperature, altitude, etc.

Table 1.8: Reference intervals for TEC in domestic animals:

Species	**Cattle**	**Goat**	**Sheep**	**Pig**	**Horse**	**Dog**	**Cat**	**Chicken**
RBC (X $10^6/\mu L$)	5-10	8-18	9-15	5-8	7-11	5.5 -8.5	5-10	2.2-4.1

Polycythemia

- Physiological polycythemia is seen in association with exercise, excessive sweating, severe vomiting, etc.
- Pathological polycythemia is seen in associated with a tissue injury (burns), polyuria, shock, diarrhea, polycythemia vera, chronic kidney diseases, carbon monoxide poisoning, lung diseases like emphysema, etc. Polycythemia vera is caused by a genetic aberration in the hemocytoblastic cells.

Oligocythemia

- Hemorrhage due to trauma, abdominal ulcers, hemorrhagic enteritis, vena cava syndrome, blood-sucking parasites (e.g., *Haemonchus* species, lice, or ticks), hemostasis defects, vessel erosion or rupture, etc.
- Oligocythemia due to destruction of erythrocytes. Hemolytic anemia is caused by blood parasites (*Babesia* species, *Theileria* species, *Trypanosoma* species, and *Sarcocystis* species), toxins, electrolyte imbalances, hypoosmolality, or autoimmune reactions, copper deficiency or chronic copper intoxication, hypophosphatemia (postparturient hemoglobinuria), water intoxication, etc.
- Less production of erythrocytes due to panleukopenia, impaired production of erythropoietin, and disorders of endocrine glands like the thyroid, adrenal, pituitary, etc.

1.9. Erythrocyte Indices or Absolute Values

Absolute values describe the characteristics of individual erythrocytes or red blood cells (RBCs). It is also known as erythrocyte indices. This value includes mean corpuscular volume (MCV), means corpuscular haemoglobin (MCH), and mean corpuscular haemoglobin concentration (MCHC). Absolute values are calculated from total RBC count, haemoglobin concentration, and PCV. These indicators aid in the diagnosis of anemia and the selection of appropriate therapies.

Procedure

- Determine the Hb concentration, total RBC count, and PCV of the blood sample as per the procedure mentioned in Chapter 1.

Calculations

a) **Mean Corpuscular Volume (MCV):** It is the average volume of the red blood cells in cubic micrometers, expressed in femtoliters (fL). One femto= 10^{-15}.

$$\text{MCV (Femtoliters or fL)} = \frac{\text{PCV in \% X 10}}{\text{RBCs number (millions /mm}^3\text{)}}$$

b) **Mean Corpuscular Haemoglobin (MCH):** It is the amount of haemoglobin content of a red blood cell expressed in picograms (pg). One pico= 10^{-12}.

$$\text{MCH (Pico grams or pg)} = \frac{\text{Haemoglobin (g/ dL) X 10}}{\text{RBC number (millions/mm}^3\text{)}}$$

c) **Mean Corpuscular Haemoglobin Concentration (MCHC):** Increased MCH does not necessarily mean that the cell is fully saturated with hemoglobin. MCHC indicates the degree of saturation of haemoglobin in the red blood cells. It is the average haemoglobin concentration per unit volume of packed red cells, expressed in percentage.

It is calculated using the haemoglobin and PCV values as follows:

$$\text{MCHC (\% or g/dL)} = \frac{\text{Haemoglobin (g/dL) X 100}}{\text{PCV (\%)}}$$

Reference values for absolute values

The erythrocyte indices or absolute values differ from species to species (Table 1.9), in animals. Most mammals, especially piglets, are born with large erythrocytes, with MVC ranging from 80-90 fL.

Table 1.9: Reference intervals for erythrocyte indices or absolute values in domestic animals:

Parameters	Dog	Cow	Horse	Pig	Sheep	Goat	Chicken
MCV (fL)	60-77	40-60	37-59	50-68	28-40	16-25	115.8
MCH (pg)	19-24	11-17	12-19	17-21	8-12	5-8	41
MCHC (g/dL)	31-34	30-36	31-39	30-34	31-34	30-36	29

Increased MCV

- The average MCV in adults varies between species of animals. If the cells are larger than normal, the cell is called a macrocyte. If smaller than normal, the cell is callled microcyte. Increased MCV is seen in associated with megaloblastic anemia, hemolytic anemia with reticulocytosis, liver disease, vitamin B_{12} or folic acid deficiency, myelodysplastic syndromes (MDS), etc. MDS is often associated with bone marrow disorders, where the body no longer makes enough healthy or normal blood cells. This disease is also known as a form of blood cancer.

Decreased MCV

- Iron deficiency anemia, thalassemia, sideroblastic anemia or sideroachrestic anemia, lead poisoning chronic infections, etc. Sideroblastic anemia is a form of anemia in which the bone marrow produces ringed sideroblasts rather than healthy RBCs.

Increased MCH

- The reference value of MCH in adult varies between species of animals. When the value is increased, the condition is described as hyperchromic. It is seen in associated with macrocytic anemia

Decreased MCH

- Microcytic, hypochromic anemia, etc

Decreased MCHC

- Spherocytes

Decreased MCHC

- Iron deficiency
- Thalassemia

1.10. Total Leucocyte Count

Leucocytes or WBCs act as a defense mechanism via cell-mediated and humoral immunity. The total leucocyte count (TLC) provides information about infections. The TLC number will vary in certain diseases. Thus, TLC aids in general health assessments, monitoring of diseases, and therapeutic actions.

Materials required

(i) Haemocytometer: The haemocytometer is a solid heavy slide with two counting chambers named Neubauer's counting chamber. This area is divided into nine (9) equal squares by triple lines. Each square has an area of 1/25 X 16 mm. WBC counts in the four corner squares.

(ii) WBC diluting pipette: The WBC diluting pipette has two markings on it: 0.5 at the bottom, and 11 at the top.

(iii) Compound microscope, sterile needle for puncturing ear, sterile cotton, etc.

Reagents and sample

- WBC diluting fluid and blood sample.

The most commonly used WBC diluting fluids are as follows:

1. **Tuerk's solution:** It contains

   a) Glacial acetic acid (1%): It destroys the erythrocytes.

   b) Gentian violet (0.3% W/V): Stains the nuclei of leucocytes.

   c) Distilled water.

2. **Toisson's fluid:** It contains

   a) Sodium sulfate 8.0 g

   b) Sodium chloride 1.0 g

   c) Glycerin 30.0 mL

   d) Distilled water 200 mL

Procedure

- Mount the haemocytometer on the mechanical stage of a microscope and focus the ruling of Neubauer's counting chamber. Put the coverslip and focus it again.

- Gently mix the vial containing anticoagulated blood.
- Draw the blood in the WBC diluting pipette up to 0.5. Remove excess blood with a fingertip, if blood is drawn beyond the 0.5 mark in the WBC diluting pipette.
- Then dilute the blood by taking WBC diluting fluid up to the upper mark above the bulb (11 in WBC). Avoid air bubbles.
- Mix the blood with the diluting fluid for about 3-5 minutes by rotating it in the palm, keeping the pipette horizontal.
- Discards 2-3 drops of diluting fluid after proper mixing.
- Wipe the tip of the pipette, then charge (one drop) the diluted blood at the edge of the coverslip at an angle of 30°. Avoid any air bubbles. Do not allow blood to flow over the coverslip. Since it will give an erroneous result.
- Allow the diluted blood to flow under the coverslip to settle the cells. Focus again at low power and adjust the illumination.
- Count the cells in the specified chamber. In the case of WBC, count the cells present in four (4) large corner squares, each containing 16 medium squares.
- The cells touching the left and upper border lines of the square can be considered for that squares, ignoring those which are falling on the right and lower border.

Calculation

1.	Area of one WBC square	$=1\text{ mm X }1\text{mm}=1\text{ mm}^2$
2.	Depth of one WBC square	$=\frac{1}{10}$ mm or 0.1 mm
3.	So, the volume of four (4) counting areas / squares is	$=\text{x }0.1\text{ mm X }1\text{ mm}^2$ $=0.4\text{ mm}^3$
4.	If the blood is taken up to the 0.5 mark of the WBC pipette, the dilution factor will be	= 20
5.	Let us assume the total number of cells counted in the 4 medium squares/ 0.4 mm^3 volume of diluted blood is	N
6.	Then, the number of WBCs present in 1 mm^3 volume of diluted blood will be	$\frac{N}{0.4}$ 0.4
8.	Therefore, total leucocytes in 1 mm^3 of undiluted blood will be	$=\frac{N}{0.4}$ X 20 (dilution factor) = n X 50

It is generally expressed as____________thousand/mm^3, or____________10^3/mm^3

Reference value of total leucocytes counts

In animals, TLC count varies greatly among species (Table 1.10). Age, exercise, emotional state, pregnancy, estrus, stage of digestion, and health status also influence the total leucocyte counts.

Table 1.10: Reference intervals for TLC in domestic animals:

Species	Cattle	Goat	Sheep	Pig	Horse	Dog	Cat	Chicken
WBC (X10^3/cu.mm)	7-10	8-10	7-10	15-22	8-11	9-13	10-15	20-30

Leucocytosis

- Physiologic leucocytosis- Stress, excitation, fear, exercise, or parturition, etc. A stress leucogram is characterized by neutrophilia, lymphocytopenia, eosinopenia, and occasionally monocytosis.
- Pathological leucocytosis-Acute bacterial infection, tissue injury (burns, surgery, and infraction), hemorrhage, inflammatory disorders, endogenous or exogenous intoxication, endocrine conditions, central nervous disorders, anaphylactic shock, leukemia, and bovine leukocyte adhesion deficiency (BLAD), etc.

Leucopenia

- Physiological leucopenia -Exposure to extreme cold. In cattle, the total number of leucocytes decreases with advancing age.
- Pathological leucopenia- viral infections, aplastic anemia, circulatory shock, peracute inflammation, metabolic disorders in cattle, rickettsiosis, bacterial septicemia, purulent splenitis, etc.

1.11. Differential Leucocyte Count

Different types of leucocytes have specific physiological functions, particularly in body defense functions. The proportion of different types of leucocytes is determined by means of a differential leucocyte count (DLC). The proportion of different types of leucocytes aids in differential diagnosis, making it an indispensable experiment for a comprehensive hematological test.

Leucocytes possess differential staining properties. Based on the staining reaction and their morphological characteristics (size and shape of the visible nucleus and staining of granules of the cytoplasm), the leucocytes are of two types: (1) granulocytes (neutrophils, eosinophils, and basophils) and (2) agranulocytes (lymphocytes and monocytes).

Materials required

- Microscopes, glass slide, staining rack, DLC counter or blood cell counter, wash bottle, etc.

Reagents and sample

- Stain, blood sample, distilled water and cedarwood oil.

1. Leishman's stain

It consists of a mixture of methylene blue (a basic stain) and eosin (an acidic stain). Methylene blue dye stains acidic cellular components blue, and eosin stains basic components of eosinophilic cytoplasmic granules red-orange.

Leishman's stain powder: 0.60 g

Acetone free methanol (Methyl alcohol): 400 mL

Mix well at intervals until the dye is completely dissolved.

2. Wright's stain

It contains methylene blue, a basic dye that stains acidic cellular components blue, and eosin, an acidic dye that stains the basic components of haemoglobin and eosinophilic cytoplasmic granules red-orange.

Wright powder : 0.1 g

Methanol : 100 mL

3. Giemsa stain

It consists of a mixture of Azure dye, eosin and methylene blue in methyl alcohol. Azure dye stains the acidic nucleus of cells blue, and eosin stains the basic components of cytoplasmic granules pink.

Giemsa powder : 3.8 g

Glycerine : 200 mL

Methanol : 312 mL

The proper dilution for working with stains is 1:10

Procedure

Preparation of blood smears

- Put a drop of either fresh or anticoagulant-mixed blood on the clean and grease-free glass slide, at least 2 mm away from the edge.

- Hold the first slide firmly with two fingers and place another slide (Spreader slide) in front of the blood drop.
- Draw the spreader slide backward till it touches the drop of blood and spread the blood across the surface between two slides.
- Any jerky movement during spreading gives an unsmooth blood smear, and the chipped edge of the spreader slide may produce some gaps in the smear.

Staining of the blood smear

1. Leishman's stain

- Select air-dried blood smears for staining.
- Keep the air-dried slides on the staining rack. The smear side should be facing upwards.
- Mark the smeared area with a wax line. Cover the smear with an undiluted staining (8 to 10 drops) solution. Leave it in an undisturbed condition for 2 minutes.
- Add double volume of distilled water or buffer solution to dilute the stain. Mix it properly by gently blowing and then keep the diluted stain at room temperature for about 15 minutes. Flush off the stain with a gentle flow of tap water for 30–60 seconds. The distilled water pH should be 6.5 for consistent results.
- Rinse the slide with water and dry it. Keeping the stained smear facing down to avoid setting off the dust on it.
- The dried smear appears bluish pink colour to the naked eye.

2. Wright's stain

- Place the air-dried smear on the slide staining rack, smear side facing upwards.
- Cover the smear with an undiluted staining solution.
- Let it allow stand for 2-3 minutes.
- Add an approximately equal amount of buffer water (pH 6.5). The diluted stain shouldn't overflow. Mix it by gently blowing, and then leave it for 5-10 minutes.
- Without disturbing the slide, flood the distilled water until the thinner parts of the film are pinkish-red in colour.

3. Giemsa stain

- Place the air-dried smear on the slide staining rack, smear side facing upwards.
- Fix the smear with a few drops of absolute alcohol for a few minutes, and then dry it in the air.
- Cover the smear with a working giemsa stain solution.
- Allow it to stand for 30-45 minutes.
- Wash the smear with distilled water and air-dry it.

Observation of stained smear under a microscope

- Select the best-stained smear for observation under a microscope. Keep the slide on the mechanical stage of a microscope and examine it first at low power and then under oil immersion at 100x magnification.
- Count at least 200 numbers of leucocytes and also count the types of leucocytes with the help of DLC counter or blood cell counter.
- Identify the different types of leucocytes based on the size and shape of the clearly visible nucleus and the stained granules in the cytoplasm of the leucocytes, as shown in Fig.1.4 and Table 1.11.
- The result will be expressed as a percentage of presence for each type of leucocyte.

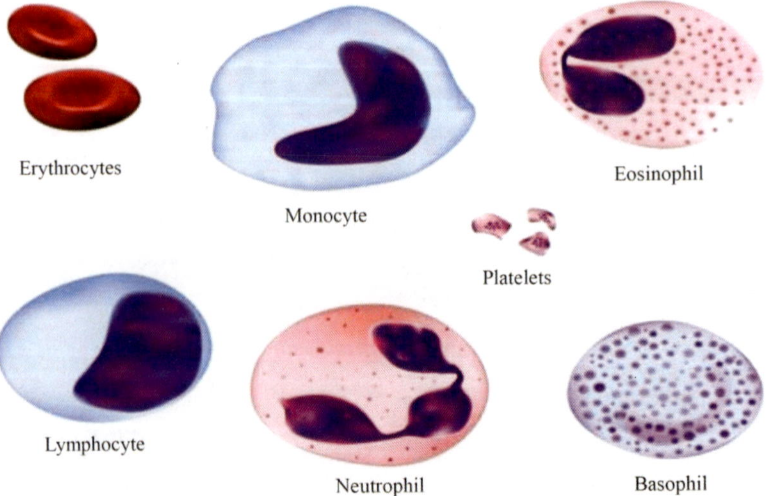

Fig. 1.4: Morphological characteristics of blood cells.

Table 1.11: Morphological and staining characteristics of different types of leucocytes:

Cell	Size(µM)	Cytoplasm	Nucleus	Location inthe smear
(A) Granulocytes				
(i) Neutrophils	10 – 12	Fine, Pinkish-blue, Diffused granules.	3 – 5 lobes, connected by chromatin filaments.	Uneven
(ii) Immature neutrophils	10 – 12	Fine, Pinkish-blue, Diffused granules.	1 – 3 lobes, connected by chromatin filaments.	Uneven
(iii) Eosinophils	10 – 15	Coarse granules contain brick-red to orange colour.	Fewer lobes often bi lobed.	Uneven
(iv) Basophils	10 – 15	Very coarse, deep purple granules in gray blue back ground.	Irregular, may be bi lobed.	Uneven
(B) Agranulocytes				
(i). Lymphocytes	7- 15	Clear light blue small cytoplasm. Large lymphocytes contain larger cytoplasmic area. Small Lymphocyte contain very small cytoplasm, Like 'ink spot'.	Single mass, deep blue, round shaped cover almost cytoplasm.	Uneven
(ii). Monocytes	15 – 25	Pale gray-blue small cytoplasm.	Single mass, kidney shaped cover almost cytoplasm.	Uneven

Reference value for differential leucocyte count

The reference value for DLC varies greatly among species (Table 1.12) in animals.

Table 1.12: Reference intervals for different leucocytes (%) in domestic animals:

Species	Cattle	Goat	Sheep	Pig	Horse	Dog	Cat	Chicken
Neutrophil (%)	25-30	35-40	25-30	30-35	50-60	65-70	55-60	25-30
Lymphocyte (%)	60-65	50-55	60-65	55-60	30-40	20-25	30-35	55-60
Monocyte (%)	5	5	5	5-6	5-6	5	5	10
Eosinophil (%)	2-5	2-5	2-5	2-5	2-5	2-5	2-5	3-8
Basophil (%)	<1	<1	<1	<1	<1	<1	<1	1-4

Neutrophilia

- Physiological causes- Exercise and epinephrine response, stress, pregnancy, lactation and parturition.

- Pathological causes- Acute pyogenic infections, tissue injury due to trauma, surgery, burn, etc. Increased number of immature neutrophils is seen in associated with bacterial infections.

Neutropenia

- Most often is seen in associated with viral infections, and chronic infections like TB, brucellosis, protozoa, fungal infections, etc.
- Aplastic anemia, corticosteroids, leukaemia, lymphoma, etc.

Note: Shift to the left is a term used to describe an increase in the number of immature neutrophils in the circulatory blood. Shifts to the right denote an increase in mature neutrophils in the circulatory blood.

Eosinophilia

- Gastrointestinal parasitic infections, allergic conditions, skin diseases, radiation therapy, poisons like copper sulphate, phosphorous, camphor, etc.

Eosinopenia

- Aplastic anemia, corticosteroids & ACTH therapy, stress, etc.

Basophilia

- Allergic conditions, chronic respiratory diseases, hematological malignancies, etc.
- Hyperlipidemia and occasionally to allergies, ulceration and parasitic infections in cattle.
- Hyperadrenocorticism in dogs.

Basopenia

- Severe septicemia, aplastic anemia, etc.

Lymphocytosis

- Chronic infections, post vaccination, autoimmune disease, physiological in calves and kittens, viral infection e.g., Hepatitis, lymphocytic leukaemia, and hypoadrenocorticism, etc.
- Chronic purulent diseases, such as hepatitis, peritonitis, pericarditis, nephritis, mastitis, or bronchopneumonia in cattle.

Lymphopenia

- Acute stress, viral or bacterial infection, immune suppression, chronic renal insufficiency, application of corticosteroids, etc.
- Radiation.

Monocytosis

- Acute stress, corticosteroid therapy, hematological malignancies, protozoa disease, viral disease, chronic infection (e.g., Tuberculosis), ACTH therapy, etc.

Monocytopenia

- Septicaemia, bone marrow suppression, etc.

1.12 Platelets count (Thrombocytes)

Platelets are specialized blood cells with an average diameter of 3 μM. These cells are colourless and spherical or rod-shaped. Avian platelets sizes range from 3 to 5 μM in width and 7 to 10 μM in length. Platelets have a life span of 8-11 days in circulating blood. Platelets perform a number of functions, including hemostasis, inflammation, tumour metastasis, wound healing, and host defence. However, the primary function is participation in hemostasis.

Platelets can be counted in two methods, viz., direct and indirect methods. In direct methods, fresh blood is diluted with Reese-Ecker fluid, which stains the platelets. These stained platelets are counted directly under a microscope using a haemocytometer, and the result is expressed as cells per mm3.

In the indirect method, blood platelets may be determined in relation to erythrocytes. For this, a thin blood smear is stained with Leishman's stain, and platelets are counted in relation to erythrocytes under a microscope. However, this method is less accurate.

Direct Method

Materials required

- Microscope, haemocytometer with coverslip, RBC diluting pipette, filter paper, cotton, syringe & needle, and spirit.

Reagents and sample

- Reese-Ecker fluid, blood, and distilled water.

Reese-Ecker fluid contains

a) Sodium citrate- 3.8 g. It acts as an anticoagulant.

b) Formaldehyde (40%)- 0.2 mL. It acts as fixative and prevent growth of fungus.

c) Brilliant cresyl blue- 0.1 g. It stains the platelets.

d) Distilled water- 100 mL.

Note: Always prepare a fresh staining solution. If prepared in advance, it should be kept in refrigerator. Further, it should be filtered just before use.

Procedure

- Draw the blood up to 0.5 marks of the RBC diluting pipette, followed by Reese - Ecker fluid up to 101 markings.
- Mix it well (blood and diluting fluid in the bulb) for about 5 minutes by rotating the pipette between the palms, keeping the pipette horizontal.
- Discard the first few drops and charge the counting chamber. The fluid is allowed to spread by capillary action between the chamber and coverslip. This is referred to as charging the Neubauer's chamber.
- Then allow it to stand for 15 minutes to settle the platelets in the counting chamber.
- Count the number of platelets (oval, round, comma-shaped, and pink-purple) in five RBC squares.

Calculation

1.	Area of one RBC square	= 1/5 X 1/5 =1/25mm^2
2.	So, area of 5 medium RBC squares	= 5 X 1/25 =1/5mm^2
3.	Hence, the volume of 5 medium RBC squares	= 1/5 X 1/10 =1/50mm^3
4.	Let us assume the total number of platelets counted in mm^3 volume of diluted blood is	N
5.	Then, the number of platelets present in 1 mm^3 volume of diluted blood will be	= N X 50 X 200 (dilutionfactor) /mm^3

Reference value for total platelets count

The reference value for platelet count in various domestic animals is shown below in Table 1.13.

Table 1.13: Reference intervals for platelet count in domestic animals:

Species	Cattle	Goat	Sheep	Pig	Horse	Dog	Cat	Chicken
Platelets (X 1000 per mm^3)	200-800	300-600	300-700	250-450	90-300	200-500	200-600	25-40

Thrombocytosis

- Physiological thrombocytosis occurs as a consequence of epinephrine-induced splenic contraction.
- Pathological thrombocytosis- Polycythemia vera
- Chronic myeloid leukaemia
- Iron deficiency anemia
- Chronic infections
- Haemorrhage

Thrombocytopenia

- Aplastic anemia
- Idiopathic thrombocytopenic purpura
- Thrombocytopenic thrombotic purpura
- Myelophthisis or bone marrow hypoplasia
- Infectious diseases such salmonellosis, leptospirosis, babesiosis, theileriosis, anaplasmosis, and BVDV infection, etc.

1.13. Erythrocyte Fragility Test

The erythrocyte membrane is non-elastic but flexible. It means that erythrocytes do not change size or shape when suspended in an isotonic solution or normal saline solution (0.9% NaCl). However, in a hypotonic solution, the cell membrane of erythrocytes ruptures, a phenomenon known as hemolysis.

The resistance of the erythrocyte cell membrane to hemolysis can be tested by reducing the concentration of NaCl in a saline solution. The degree of vulnerability to hemolysis in a hypotonic solution varies significantly between species in animals. It also relies on the size of the cells. As a result, large-sized canine erythrocytes are more resistant than smaller-sized goat erythrocytes. Some diseases have different levels of susceptibility.

Materials required

- Test tubes
- Test tube rack

- Glass marker
- Pipette
- Syringe with needle (2 mL)
- Cotton
- Pasteur pipette

Reagents and sample

- Blood (freshly drawn blood, preferably heparinized blood samples).
- Normal saline solution (1.0%).
- Distilled water.

Procedure

- Arrange the test tubes in the rack serially from 1 to 16 after marking them with a marker pen.
- Add 1.0 % NaCI solution and the required quantity of distilled water to all test tubes using a measuring pipette as shown in the table below.
- Mix the solution well by gently shaking.
- Put a drop of blood into each test tube with a Pasteur pipette and mix them by gently shaking.
- Allow the tubes to stand undisturbed for 1 hour. The degree of hemolysis is then measured against a white sheet of paper held behind them. Because tube no. 1 contains isotonic normal saline, there will be no hemolysis. In tube no. 16, which contains distilled water with zero tonocity, there will be total hemolysis. As a result, tubes 1 and 16 serve as controllers.
- Where there is no hemolysis, the erythrocytes settle down, leaving the clear-normal saline at the top. If there is some hemolysis, the solution is tinged red, with a few cells at the bottom. The degree of hemolysis can be measured by colour of the solution and the number of erythrocytes at the bottom. Hemolysis increases with decreasing tonicity.
- Take note of the minimum and maximum strengths of the NaCl solution, where mild and complete hemolysis has occurred, respectively.

Note: Osmotic fragility begins at 0.45 to 0.50 g/dL or% and ends at 0.34 g/dL or%. Erythrocyte fragility tests, like haematological indices, are influenced by a variety of parameters, including breed, age, reproductive state, season, and environmental conditions. This value is also affected by factors such as sample collection and preparation as well as transport time.

Tube No	**1**	**2**	**3**	**4**	**5**	**6**	**7**	**8**	**9**	**10**	**11**	**12**	**13**	**14**	**15**	**16**
% NaCl (mL)	4.25	4.00	3.75	3.50	3.25	3.00	2.75	2.50	2.25	2.00	1.75	1.50	1.25	1.00	0.50	0.00
D. water (mL)	0.75	1.00	1.25	1.50	1.75	2.00	2.25	2.50	2.75	3.00	3.25	3.50	3.75	4.00	4.50	5.00
Tonicity	0.85	0.80	0.75	0.70	0.65	0.60	0.55	0.50	0.45	0.40	0.35	0.30	0.25	0.20	0.10	0.00

Increased osmotic fragility

- Pathological causes - Hereditary spherocytosis, congenital haemolytic anemia, etc.

Decreased osmotic fragility

- Iron deficiency anemia, sickle cell anemia, thalassaemia, etc.

1.14. Specific Gravity of Blood

Specific gravity is defined as the ratio of the weight of a volume of blood to the weight of the same volume of water. The specific gravity of blood is directly related to the volume and gravity of RBCs, their haemoglobin concentration, plasma proteins, and the balance of fluid exchanges between blood and tissue. Specific gravity of blood or plasma can be evaluated indirectly with copper sulfate ($CuSO_4$) solution. It is based on the property of plasma proteins that form a copper propionate with copper sulfate and a pellicle around the blood drop and prevent its disintegration.

Materials required

- Pipette, test tube, beaker, and measuring cylinder.

Reagents and sample

- Copper sulfate solution, blood sample and distilled water.

The specific gravity of copper sulfate stock solution is 1.10, which contains 170g of $CuSO_4$ and 100 mL of distilled water. This solution has to be filtered and stored. Prepare a working solution with a specific gravity of 1.020 to 1.070.

Procedure

- Take seven beakers and number them from 1 to 7. Add a working $CuSO_4$ solution in the beaker serially.
- Add a drop of blood to each $CuSO_4$ solution in beakers by using a dropper very slowly. EDTA is the anticoagulant of choice for blood collection to determine the specific gravity of the blood.
- Then observe the reaction. The blood droplets will sink if the specific gravity of the blood is greater than that of the solution, and float if the specific gravity of the blood is less than that of the solution.

Note: The specific gravity of plasma can be determined in the same way as that of blood.

Reference value of specific gravity of blood

The specific gravity of the blood is mostly determined by the plasma protein concentration. The Table-1.14 shows the reference value of specific gravity in several domestic animals.

Table 1.14: Reference intervals for the specific gravity of blood in domestic animals:

Species	Cattle	Goat	Sheep	Pig	Horse	Dog	Cat	Chicken
Specific Gravity	1.046-1.061	1.036-1.051	1.041-1.061	1.035-1.055	1.046-1.059	1.045-1.052	1.045-1.057	1.042 -1.049

Increased specific gravity of blood

- Physiological polycytemia, polycythemia vera, severe dehydration due to excessive vomiting & diarrhoea, and hemoconcentration due to plasma loss such as in burns.

Decreased specific gravity of blood

- Anemia, pregnancy, renal disease, prolongs glucocorticoid therapy, etc.

1.15. Viscosity of Blood and Plasma

Blood viscosity refers to the 'thickness' of the blood, or its resistance to flow normally. The number (and volume) of erythrocytes and the concentration of plasma proteins such as fibrinogen, α1-globulins, α2-globulins, β-globulins, and γ-globulins influence blood viscosity. A viscometer can be used to determine the viscosity of blood. It is determined by comparing the time required to flow a blood sample through a viscometer against the time required to flow the same amount of distilled water.

Materials required

- Viscometer, pipettes, pipette tips and stopwatch.

Reagents and sample

- Blood, plasma and distilled water.

Procedure

- Attach the rubber tube with a pinch cook to the viscometer and draw distilled water up to the mark above the bulb. Close the pinch cock.
- Fix the viscometer vertically. Wipe the tip.
- Release the pinch cock while starting the stopwatch. When the meniscus reaches the mark below the bulb, stop the watch.

- Take note of how long it takes for the water to flow out.
- Repeat with blood and plasma in a dry viscometer. Take note of the time required for blood and plasma separately.

Calculation

- Viscosity of blood: Blood time X specific gravity (1.06) / water time.
- Viscosity of plasma: Plasma time X specific gravity (1.06) / water time.

Increased viscosity of blood and plasma

- Physiological polycytemia in high altitudes
- Polycythemia vera
- Ccongestive heart failure
- Jaundice
- Severe dehydration due to excessive vomiting and diarrhoea
- Hemoconcentration due to plasma loss such as in burns

Decreased viscosity of blood and plasma

- It is commonly seen in associated with anemia, edema, etc.

1.16. Blood Grouping

Blood transfusions can save an individual's life. However, incompatibility between donor and recipient blood may result in intravascular hemolysis and other clinical complications in the recipient animal. In certain incompatible blood transfusions, IgM is naturally produced against red blood cells. This is why blood must be typed and cross-matched to avoid adverse effects in recipient animals induced by serum antibodies.

The genetically regulated surface antigens on red blood cells determine blood groups. Blood can be divided into groups based on the presence or lack of specific types of glycol proteins on the surface of red blood cells. Red blood cells have many antigens (molecular weight of 20,000 to 30,000) on their cell membrane that are glycoproteins in nature. In 1990, Landsteiner first discovered the human ABO blood grouping system. There are two forms of agglutinogens: agglutinogen-A and agglutinogen-B, as well as two types of agglutinins: agglutinin-a or Anti-A and agglutinin-b or Anti-B. The precise function of blood group antigens is unknown. Also, Rh agglutinogen is found in red blood cells in human's blood. 'D' is the most important subgroup among

C, D, and E. If 'D' agglutinogen is present in the red blood cell membrane, the group of blood is R+ ve; if 'D' agglutinogen is lacking, the group of blood is Rh-ve.

Contrary to humans, the classification of blood groups in animals varies greatly from species to species. The blood groups of many domestic animals are shown in Table 1.15 below.

Table 1.15: Blood group types in domestic animals:

S.No	Species	No. of blood group	Blood group system and blood Type	Iso-antibodies
1	Canine	13	Blood grouping in dogs is based on erythrocyte antigens (DEA), Kai, and Dal antigens. DEA 1, 3, 4, 5, and 7 blood types are recognized, internationally.	Occasionally
2	Feline	2	AB blood group system. Types of blood include A and B. The blood group AB is rare.	Rare
3	Equine	7	Blood types: A, C, D, K, P, Q, and U.	Rare
4	Bovine	11	Blood types: A, B, C, F, J, L, M, R, S, T andZ.	None
5	Ovine	7	Blood types:A, B, C, D, M, R, and X.	None
6	Caprine	6	Blood types: A, B, C, M, R and X.	None
7	Porcine	16	-	Rare

Methods of blood grouping

1. Card agglutination (CARD) method
2. Immunochromatographic cartridge (CHROM) method
3. Gel-based agglutination (GEL) method
4. Slide agglutination (SLIDE) method
5. Tube agglutination (TUBE) method
6. Alloantibody testing

The slide agglutination (SLIDE) method is the most frequent and easiest to demonstrate. This test is based on the agglutination reaction of RBC surface antigens and antibodies (anti-sera) produced against that specific surface antigen. ABO antibodies in serum are produced naturally. The basic biology of the link between ABO antigens and antibodies in the human ABO blood grouping system is shown in Table 1.16 below.

Table 1.16: Basic biochemistry of the ABO blood grouping system:

Blood group	Antigen / agglutinogen present on the surface of RBCs	Antibodies present in the serum
A	A Antigen	Anti-B
B	B Antigen	Anti-A
AB	A Antigen and B Antigen	None
O	Nil / None	Anti-A and Anti-B

Materials required

- Lancet, spirit, cotton, blood, glass slide, glass rod for mixing and microscope.

Reagents and sample

- Monoclonal antiserum for A, B &Rh factors, and blood samples.

Procedure

- Take two grease-free glass slides. Then, using a marker pen, mark one side as A, B, and Rh on one glass slide.
- Put one drop of antiserum A, B, and Rh factors on a slide's marked area.
- Add one drop of a test blood sample to each antiserum.
- Mix the blood with the reagent (antiserum) using a clean stick. Then allow it to stand for 2-3 minutes.
- Spread the mixture evenly over an area of 15mm.
- Rotate the slide gently to and fro while looking for agglutination with your naked eyes. The agglutination reaction can be observed using a microscope.
- Record the results.

Interpretation

- The presence or absence of RBC agglutination reveals the individual's blood group, as indicated below:

Antiserum A	Antiserum B	Agglutinogen on RBCs	Agglutinin in plasma	Blood group
+	-	A	Anti-B	A
-	+	B	Anti-A	B
+	+	AB	Nili	AB
-	-	Nil	Anti-A and Anti-B	O

Note: The test should be performed on fresh blood obtained in a vial without anticoagulants.

Table 1.17: Reference intervals for biochemical constituents of blood in domestic animals:

Variables	Domestic animals						
	Cattle	**Dog**	**Horse**	**Goat**	**Pig**	**Sheep**	**Chicken**
Albumin (g/dL)	3.0-3.8	3.4-4.4	2.8-3.8	3.7-4.5	3.2-4.0	3.5-4.5	1.6-2.0
Globulin (g/dL)	3.6-4.4	2.2-3.2	2.8-3.8	2.4-3.2	3.4-4.0	2.5-3.5	2.3-3.3
Fibrinogen (g/ dL)	0.2-0.5	0.1-0.4	0.2-0.4	0.2-0.5	0.2-0.4	0.2-0.4	-
BUN (mg/dL)	10-30	10-30	20-40	10-28	8-24	8-20	0.4-1.0
Uric acid (mg/ dL)	0.1-2	0.1-1.5	0.5-1	0.3-1	0.1-2	0.1-2	1-2
Creatinine (mg/ dL)	1-2	1-2	1-2	1-2	1-2.5	1-2	1-2
Direct bilirubin (mg/dL)	0-0.3	0.06-0.1	0-0.4	-	0-0.3	0-0.3	-
Glucose (mg/ dL)	40-80 80-120(calf)	70-120	60-110	40-75 80-120 (Kid)	80-120	40-80 80-120 (Lamb)	130-270
Cholesterol (mg/dL)	80-180	120-250	75-150	80-160	60-200	60-150	125-200
Calcium (mEq/L)	4.5-6.0	4.5-6.0	4.5-6.5	4-5-6.0	4.5-6.5	4.5-6.0	4.5-6.0 8.5-19.5 lying hen)
Phosphorus (mEq/L)	2-7	2-6	2-6	2-6	3-6	2-7	3-6
Magnesium (mEq/L)	1.5-2.5	1.5-2.0	1.5-2.5	2-3	2-3	1.8-2.3	-
Potassium (mEq/L)	3.9-5.8	3.7-5.8	2.5-5.0	3.5-6.7	4.4-6.7	3.9-5.4	4.6-4.7
Sodium (mEq/L)	132-152	141-155	132-152	142-155	135-150	139-182	151-161
Chloride (mEq/L)	97-111	100-115	99-109	99-110	94-106	95-105	119-130

2

Cardiovascular System: Measuring Cardiovascular Response

2.0. Introduction

The cardiovascular system is comprised of the heart and blood vessels (arteries, capillaries, and veins). The heart pumps blood to blood vessels which allow blood to flow throughout the body. Both heart and blood vessels are work together to keep the blood circulating, ensuring the interchange of O_2, CO_2, electrolytes, and nutrients between the blood and the tissue fluids & cells, and removing waste products from the body via the excretory system.

The purpose of the study of the cardiovascular system is aimed at understand the pathophysiology of the heart and vascular system. A physical examination, arterial blood pressure, and electrocardiography are routinely employed to examine the cardiovascular system. The physical examination of the heart includes palpation, percussion, and auscultation.

2.1. Heart Sounds

The closure of cardiac valves during the cardiac cycle produces heart sounds, which are heard with a stethoscope. Auscultation of the heart is performed to determine normal and abnormal heart sounds, heart rate, rhythm, and intensity. Abnormal heart sound indicates the presence of cardiac disease. Auscultation of heart sounds is done with the help of a stethoscope. It is a valuable first-line tool to detect heart pathology. In veterinary medicine, phonocardiography is used to detect cardiac murmurs, where factors such as uncooperative patients, rapid heart rates, and panting or purring decrease the sensitivity and accuracy of cardiac auscultation.

Materials required

- Stethoscope and service crate (in case of large animals).

Procedure

- Restrain the animal gently in a quiet room or service crate (in the case of a large animal), and a standing position is preferred.
- Place the stethoscope (chest piece) between the fourth and fifth left intercostal space over each heart valve (pulmonic–aortic–tricuspid–mitral valves) and earpieces into the ear canals of the observer. The anatomic location of the valve areas is influenced by the species, breed, chest conformation, and heart size.
- Then listen carefully to evaluate the heart sounds. The first and second heart sounds are sharp and loud and are referred to as 'LUB' and 'DUB', respectively. A third or fourth heart sound could be heard. When examining heart sounds, the first and second heart sounds are often employed as a reference platform for the auscultation of murmurs and aberrant or abnormal heart sounds.

Abnormal heart sound

Abnormal heart sounds are classified as (a) cardiac murmurs, (b) splitting of heart sounds, (c) systolic clicks (d) cardiac gallops, (e) muffled heart sounds, and (f) audible arrhythmias.

(a) Heart mummer sound – It is seen in associated with abnormalities in the size of vascular or valve orifices, abnormal communications, and alterations in blood velocity and viscosity.

(b) Splitting heart sound- Pulmonary hypertension is usually seen due to heartworm disease, pulmonic stenosis, or right bundle branch block or in normal dogs during inspiration. Splitting heart sounds are considered normal in large-breed dogs.

(c) Systolic clicks- Pulmonary stenosis and pulmonary hypertension.

(d) Cardiac gallop - Hypertrophic cardiomyopathy, and galloping horse.

(e) Muffled heart sound- Disorders such as pericardial and pleural effusion, diaphragmatic hernias, thoracic neoplasia, obesity, and hypothyroidism.

(f) Audible arrhythmias–Arrhythmias include an abnormal heart rate, an irregular cadence, the irregular intensity of the heart sounds, extra or absent heart sounds or the splitting of the first and second heart sounds. It is also seen in associated with sinus arrhythmia and atrial fibrillation.

2.2. Pulse Rate

The arterial pulse is the rhythmic expansion of an artery due to blood transport during each systole of the heart. The pulse rate is the number of times the artery wall rises and falls each minute. The pulse rate reflects the complicated hemodynamic interaction of stroke volume, heart rate, aortic compliance, and peripheral vascular tone. As a result, measuring pulse rate helps understand the health of the cardiovascular system and also aids in disease prognosis.

Procedure

- Restrain the animal gently in a quiet room or service crate (in the case of a large animal), and a standing position is preferred.
- Place the tip of your index or middle finger on the artery to feel the pulse. The pulse rate should be recorded from a superficial artery, which varies for different animals as shown below in Table 2.1.
- Count the number of arterial wall rises and falls for at least 30 seconds or one minute. While taking the pulse, consider the pulse rate, rhythm, and quality.

Table 2.1: Suitable sites for recording pulse rate in domestic animals:

Animals	**Sites and locations**
Horse, Donkey, Mule	External maxillary artery. This artery is located on the medial aspect of the ventral border of mandible.
Cattle, Buffalo, and Yak	Middle coccygeal artery. This artery is located on the ventral aspect of the tail. 8-10 cm away from the base of the tail.
Sheep, Goat, Calf, Pig, Dog, and Cat	Femoral artery. This artery is located in the inguinal region on the medial aspect of thigh.

Pulse rate of domestic animals

In animals, the reference value for pulse rate varies from species to species. Also pulse rates vary according to age, pregnancy, lactation, enthusiasm, meal ingestion, rumination (in ruminant animals), and environmental temperature. The Table 2.2 below shows the reference value for the pulse rate of in domestic animals.

Table 2.2: Reference value for pulse rate in domestic animals:

Species	**Cattle**	**Horse**	**Sheep**	**Pig**	**Dog (Large)**	**Dog (Small)**	**Goat**
Pulse rate/minute	45-60	33-41	60-70	60-90	70-90	90-120	60-70

2.3. Arterial Blood Pressure

Blood pressure (BP) is defined as the force exerted by flowing blood against any unit area of artery walls. Stephen Hales measured BP in horses first during the early 18th century. Arterial BP is required for normal and sufficient oxygen delivery to tissues or cells. Monitoring arterial BP gives crucial information about cardiovascular status and may aid in the formulation of a treatment strategy.

Method of estimation of blood pressure

BP can be measured by two methods

(A) Direct method

(B) Indirect method

2.3.A. Direct Method

Arterial blood pressure is monitored directly using a pressure transducer by introducing a catheter into an animal's artery. The catheter is connected to a pressure transducer. This method provides for continuous measurement of systolic, diastolic, and mean pressures, as well as continuous invasive monitoring of arterial blood pressure and variations in blood pressure. This method is the most accurate way to monitor arterial blood pressure.

Materials required

- Arterial catheter and pressure transducer.

Reagents

- 0.9% NaCl and sprit.

Procedure

- Restrain the animal gently in sternal or lateral recumbency.
- Select a peripheral artery for catheter insertion. The dorsal pedal artery, superficial palm arch, brachial artery, dorsal pedal artery, digital artery, coccygeal artery, and jugular artery are preferred for animals.
- Clip the hair coat over the sleeted artery and wet it with spirit or alcohol.
- Insert the artery catheter and connect it to a pressure transducer monitoring device.

- Then, at one end of the pressure transducer monitoring system, connect a 20 mL heparinized tubing bag of 0.9% NaCl. The basic purpose is to maintain a fluid bag pressure greater than the patient's systolic pressure, which prevents arterial blood from back flowing into the monitoring system. The pressure transducer translates "pressure changes" in the artery into an electrical signal that is displayed on the pressure transducer's monitor.

2.3. B. Indirect Method

This method is based on obstructing blood flow through a large artery by applying air pressure through a rubber bag wrapped around the animal's limb or tail. The blood pressure is then measured using one of two methods: palpation or auscultation. Both mercury manometers and aneroid barometers can be used to measure blood pressure.

Materials required

1. **Sphygmomanometer**

   The sphygmomanometer is consisted of the following parts -

   a. Inflatable cuff: An armlet made up of a rubber bag encased in non-distensible silk fabric.

   b. Pressure bulb: Made up of rubber with a screw valve for releasing the pressure.

   c. Manometer: This may be either mercurial or aneroid. It measures the pressure developed inside the cuff by the bulb.

2. Stethoscope: It consists of a chest piece, tubing, and earpieces.

Palpatory method

- Palpate the most suitable superficial artery for measuring blood pressure. The choice of the artery for measurement of BP varies from species to species in animals, as shown below in Table 2.3.
- Wrap the inflatable cuff around the selected superficial artery of the leg or tail.
- Position the manometer such that the centre of the mercury column or aneroid dial is at eye level and easily visible to the observer and the tubing from the cuff is unobstructed.

- Then, slowly inflate the cuff with the pressure bulb beyond the desired systolic BP level. Simultaneously, feel the arterial pulse distal to the occlusion during cuff pressure inflation and deflation.
- Take note of the pressure at which the pulse disappears (systolic pressure) and reappears (diastolic pressure) during deflation.

Auscultatory method

- Palpate the most suitable superficial artery for measuring blood pressure. The choice of the artery for measurement of BP varies from species to species in animals, as shown below in Table 2.3.
- Place the stethoscope (chest piece) over the artery and the earpieces in the observer's ear canals.
- Set the manometer so that the centre of the mercury column or aneroid dial is at eye level, easily visible to the observer, and that the tubing from the cuff is clear.
- Then, slowly inflate the cuff with the pressure bulb until the superficial artery is totally blocked by the cuff pressure. When inflating the cuff, no sound is heard at some point, indicating that the artery is completely blocked.
- Unscrew the valve to reduce the pressure while listening for the Korotkoff noises, as illustrated in Fig. 2.1. Note the pressure level's appearance with distinct, clear, and tapping noises (Phase-I), followed by the final disappearing sounds (Phase-V) when the pressure in the cuff lowers.
- Record the systolic (Phase-I) and diastolic pressure (Phase-V).

Table 2.3: The most suitable superficial artery for measurement of blood pressure in domestic animals:

Animals	**Target artery for indirect measurement of BP**
Horse	Middle coccygeal artery at the base of the tail. Median or dorsal interosseous artery on the forelegs.
Dog	Brachial artery on forelegs.Femoral artery in hind leg.
Cattle and Buffalo	Middle coccygeal artery at the base of the tail.

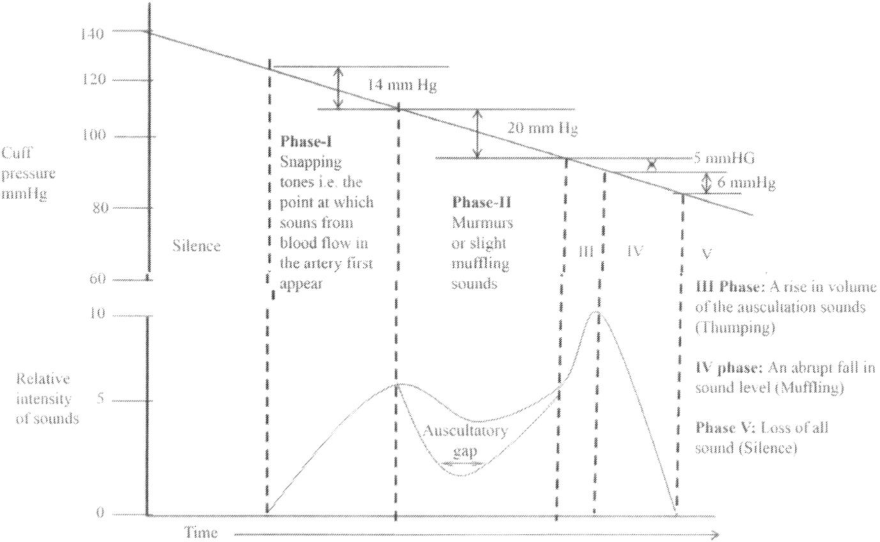

Fig. 2.1: Illustration of characteristics of the auscultatory method of measuring blood pressure.

Blood pressure of domestic animals

In animals, the reference value for blood pressure varies between species. The blood pressure of animals is shown in Table 2.4 below.

Table 2.4: Reference intervals for blood pressure of domestic animals:

Species	Cow	Horse	Sheep	Pig	Dog	Cat	Giraffe
Blood pressure (mm Hg)	140/95	130/95	140/90	140/80	120/70	140/90	260/160

Hypertension

- The development of hypertension is a result of complex interactions between endocrine, renal, vascular, and autonomic nervous systems. The development of hypertension is reared in veterinary patients compared to humans. Hypertension is generally associated with vasoconstriction, renal diseases, hyperthyroidism, hyperadrenocorticism, and endocrinopathies, etc.

Hypotension

- The basic mechanisms that lead to hypotension are decreased vascular tone, vascular dilatation, decreased cardiac output, and hypovolemia. Hypotension is seen in associated with certain diseases, particularly those related to anaphylaxis, blood loss, anemia, neoplasia, sepsis, acidosis, abnormality of heart, etc.

2.4 Recording of Electrocardiogram (ECG)

Electrocardiography (ECG or EKG) is a graphical representation of the heart's electric potential during a heartbeat. It is a non-invasive method of assessing cardiac function, such as heart rate, rhythm, amplitudes, and conduction. It is most often used to diagnose heart conduction disorders and cardiac diseases such as arrhythmias (other than sinus arrhythmias in dogs), myocardial infarction, pharmacological effects, etc.

The electrical activities of the heart are circulated through bodily fluids and detected by surface electrodes placed at specified places on the skin of the ECG machine. A typical ECG wave is made up of a "P" wave, a "QRS" complex, and a "T" wave. The "QRS" complex is frequently made up of three distinct waves: the "Q" wave, the "R" wave, and the "S" wave. The "P" wave represents the right and left atria's depolarization. The "QRS" complex represents depolarization of the ventricle. The "Q" wave, which is represented by septal depolarization, is the first phase of ventricular depolarization. Ventricular repolarization is shown by the "T" wave.

Materials required

- ECG machine, Electrocardiograph leads system (electrodes), ECG recording paper and ECG jelly.

ECG machine: A device that records the electrical activity of the heart.

Electrocardiograph-leads system: A lead system is made up of two wires and electrodes that are connected to an electrocardiograph. The following lead systems are employed for electrocardiogram recording:

1. Bipolar leads.
2. Unipolar leads.

1. Bipolar leads

Bipolar leads are also referred to as triaxial leads. Willem Einthoven invented the bipolar triaxial lead system, as well as the P-QRS-T terminology that characterizes the ECG wave complex, in the early twentieth century. It contains lead-I, lead-II, and lead-III. In bipolar electrocardiography, a lead is attached to two areas of the body by electrodes, and the potential difference between the two electrodes is recorded. Bipolar lead placement is shown in Table 2.5 and Fig. 2.2a.

Table 2.5: Appropriate site for placement of bipolar leads in animals:

Lead	**Placement position**	
	Positive (+Ve) electrodes	**Negative (-Ve) electrodes**
Lead-I	Left foreleg	Right foreleg
Lead-II	Left hind leg	Right foreleg
Lead-III	Left hind leg	Left foreleg

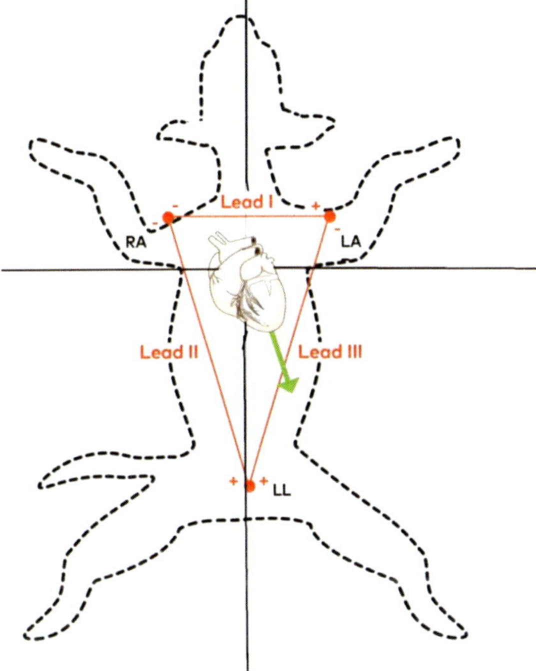

Fig. 2.2a: Illustration of placement of bipolar leads and Einthoven's triangle.

2. Unipolar leads: Unipolar leads are classified into two distinct types:

- Augmented unipolar limb leads.
- Unipolar chest leads or Unipolar precordial leads.

*Augment unipolar limb leads:*The recording from two electrodes is summed and then compared with the recording from the third electrode in augmented unipolar limb leads.The leads are represented by the letters aVR, aVL, and aVF, where a=augmented, V=voltage, R=right foreleg/arm, L=left foreleg/arm, and F=left leg/hind leg. The lead placement is shown in Table 2.6.

Table 2.6: Appropriate sites for placement of augmented unipolar limb leads in animals:

Lead	Placement position	
	Positive (+Ve) electrodes	**Negative (-Ve) electrodes**
aVR	Right foreleg	Left foreleg and left hind leg
aVL	Left foreleg	Right foreleg and left hind leg
aVF	Left hind leg	Right foreleg and left foreleg

Unipolar chest leads: There are six chest leads in this lead system, which are denoted V1, V2, V3, V4, V5, and V6. The lead placement is shown in Table 2.7.

Table 2.7: Appropriate sites for placement of unipolar chest leads in animals:

Lead	Placement position
V_1	Right 4th intercostal space near sternum
V_2	Left 4th intercostal space near sterna border
V_3	Midway between V_2 and V_4
V_4	Left 5th intercostal space at mid clvicular line
V_5	Left anterior axillary line in the level of V_4
V_6	Left mid axillary line in the level of V_4 and V_5

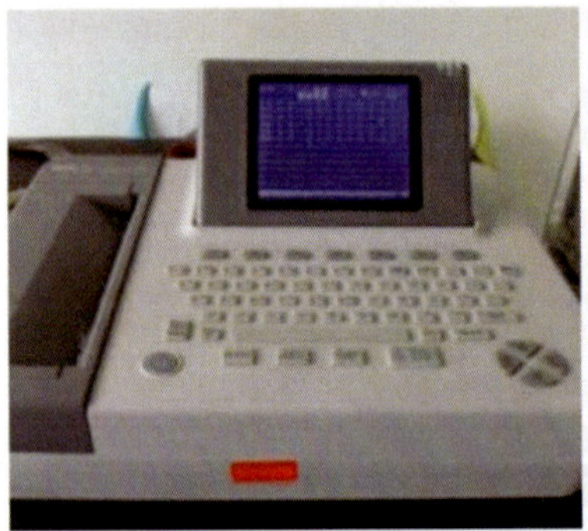

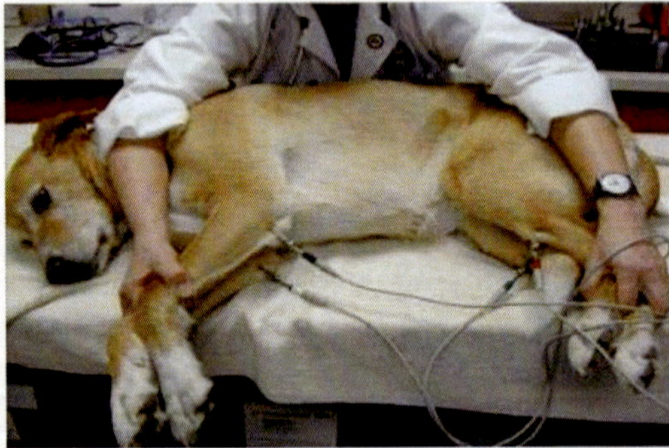

Fig. 2.2b: Illustration of the Electrocardiography of a patient placed in right lateral recumbency in dogs.

Procedure

- Position the animal on an insulated tolly table. Ideally, the animals should be immobilized in an area that is as quiet and distraction-free as possible. Right lateral recumbency is preferred in dogs and cats, as shown in Fig.2.2b.
- Prepare the site for the placement of electrodes by clipping the hair and shaving, if required.

- Connect each electrode to the appropriate limb as illustrated in Fig. 2.2b using a contact plate fastened or clamped to the limb after applying the ECG jelly. Ideally, the electrodes should be placed distal to the elbows and hock joints.
- Turn on the instrument and let it calibrate in either auto or manual mode. The heat of the stylus should be properly adjusted so that it leaves a good mark on the ECG recording paper. In addition, the ECG recording paper speed should be set to 25 mm/second.
- Remove the ECG paper strip from the device once the recording is complete to analyze or interpret it.

ECG interpretations

The ECG is interpreted using the following measurements:

- P-wave amplitude and duration.
- P-R interval.
- QRS complex duration.
- R-wave amplitude.
- T- wave amplitude and duration.
- Q-T interval.
- P-R segment.
- S-T segment.

ECG specific measurements

A normal ECG-specific measurement interval and heart rate differ between species in animals. The average heart rate and reference value for ECG intervals of various domestic animals are shown in Table 2.8 below.

Table 2.8: Average heart rate and normal baseline values of ECG in domestic animals:

Species	Average heart rate	Intervals in seconds		
		PR	QRS	QT
Cattle	70 (48 – 84)	0.18	0.09	0.39
Horse	35 (28 - 40)	0.30	0.11	0.52
Swine	100 (70-120)	0.13	0.06	0.32
Sheep/goat	100 (72-120)	0.13	0.04	0.28
Dog	100 (70-120)	0.10	0.04	0.06

Abnormal ECG values

- Absences of the "P"-wave in the ECG wave indicate several dysrhythmias, including atrial fibrillation and atrial standstill.
- A prolonged P-R interval suggests atrioventricular delay and is termed first-degree AV blocking (AV block). While only the "P" wave is blocked, i.e., it does not result in a "QRS" complex, the rhythm is termed a second-degree AV block.
- If the "P" wave and "QRS" complexes are completely unrelated, the rhythm is termed a third-degree AV block.
- S-T elevation is seen in a association with myocardial infarction.
- S-T depression is seen in association with myocardial ischaemia.
- A tall "T" wave is seen in association with Hyperkalemia.
- A prominent "T" wave is seen in association with myocardial hypoxia, and interventricular conduction disturbances.
- A biphasic "T" wave is seen in association with ischaemia and hypokalemia.
- Shortening of the Q-T interval is seen in association with hypercalcemia,
- hyperkalemia, or digoxin therapy.
- Prolonged Q-T intervals are associated with conditions such as bradycardia, electrolyte imbalance, and CNS disturbance.

3

Digestive System Enzyme Activity and Ruminoreticular Microenvironment Evaluations

3.0. Introduction

The digestive system and its auxiliary organs main functions include digestion and the absorption of nutrients required for cell metabolic processes. Digestion is the mechanical and chemical or enzymatic breakdown of large nutritional macromolecules into simpler molecules that cells can absorb. It takes place in the aqueous milieu of the digestive system and is secreted by the salivary glands, stomach and mucosal glands, pancreas, and liver.

Digestive enzymes are secreted almost throughout the digestive tract. Salivary enzymes such as lingual lipase and α-amylase initiate the breakdown of fat and carbohydrates in the mouths of young animals (e.g., calves) and omnivores (e.g., rats, pigs, and humans).The optimum pH for oral digestion is 6.7 (6.2-7.6).

The gastric juice contains pepsinogen, HCI, and intrinsic factors. The pepsinogen enzyme is secreted by the stomach's chief cell. Pepsinogen is converted to pepsin at acidic pH ranges of 2.0 to 3.5 and initiates the digestion of proteins in the stomach of monogastric animals. Also, the stomach's parietal cells secrete HCI and intrinsic factors. Cyanocobalamin, is a synthetic form of vitamin B_{12} requires an intrinsic factor in ruminants to be absorbed. The abomasum of young ruminants secretes proteolytic enzymes such as rennin or chymosin. Rennin acts on milk at a pH of 6.5.

Pancreatic enzymes are amylases, lipases, and proteases. The pH of these enzymes should be about 7-9. In the presence of a protein colipase and bile acids, pancreatic lipase hydrolyzes triglycerides to fatty acids and monoglycerides in the intestines. Proteases, which hydrolyze protein peptide bonds, include elastase, gelatinase, chymotrypsin, and trypsin. Chymotrypsin and trypsin are both secreted as inactive proenzymes known as chymotrypsinogen and trypsinogen, respectively. Enterokinase in the duodenum activates these proenzymes. Most proteins are broken down into dipeptides by activated enzymes. Furthermore, the activity of these enzymes continues within the brush border of the intestines. Disaccharidases, which hydrolyze carbohydrates include maltase, lactase, isomaltase, and trehalase. Glucose is the end product of carbohydrate digestion, which is absorbed into the bloodstream through the intestinal wall.

Bile is secreted by the liver and aids in digestion and absorption of fats in the small intestine. It is comprised of water, cholesterol, bile acids (cholic acids), phospholipids, and bile pigments (bilirubin and biliverdin), etc.

In ruminant animals, the foremost step of digestion is microbial fermentation. Microorganisms of the rumen and reticulum secrete enzymes such as amylase, β-glucanase, maltase, lipase, cellulase, pectinase, protease, xylanase, tannase, etc. for microbial digestion in ruminant animals. Plant cell wall polymers are digested by the enzymes cellulase, pectinase, protease, and xylanase. Amylase is primarily responsible for breaking down starches into glucans and maltose. β-glucanase and maltase hydrolyze glucans and maltose into glucose molecules, which are subsequently available for microbes or absorption by the host. The end products of microbial fermentative digestion in ruminant animals are VFAs, short-chain branching VFAs, lactate, polyunsaturated fatty acids, minimal glucose, hydrogenated fatty acids, and gas (CO_2, CH_4, N_2, H_2S, and H_2).

The host reticulorumen environment must ensure the following conditions for optimal microbial fermentative digestion to occur:

1. A neutral rumen pH of 5.6-6.8 is preferable.
2. The rumen temperature must be maintained at or around 37°C.
3. The rumen fluid's ionic strength must be maintained 285 mOs or less than plasma osmolality (300 mOsm).
4. The oxidation-reduction potential (ORP) or redox potential must be maintained between -250 and -450.
5. The substrate for fermentation must be continuously provided to the rumen.
6. VFAs, gases, and solid or indigestible waste products must be eliminated from the rumen.

Therefore, the purposes of the examination of the digestive system are to know about the health status of the digestive system, the rumen ecosystem, and digestion trials for the evaluation of the nutritive value of feeds.

3.1. Counting of Rumen Motility

Reticulorumen contracts one to three times every five minutes. In general, two reticulorumen motility patterns are described and they are:

- Primary or mixing contraction (Primary cycle).
- Secondary or eructation contraction (Secondary cycle).

Primary (Mixing) contraction

Primary contraction begins with a biphasic or double reticular contraction, followed by monophasic contractions of the dorsal and ventral ruminal sacs. This contraction keeps the rumen contents properly mixed, allowing for efficient microbial or fermentative digestion in ruminants. It also aids in regurgitation and controls the passage of ingesta from the reticulo-rumen to the omasum.

Secondary (Eructation) contraction

Secondary contractions occur soon following primary contractions. This contraction moves the gases in the ruminal sac towards the cardia in preparation for eructation.

The reticulum experiences triphasic contractions during rumination. It is a more powerful additional contraction that occurs before the regular biphasic contraction. During rumination, the primary wave of the ventral sac is missing, but there are powerful and sustained ventral sac movements as a secondary wave.

Method of recording rumen motility

A. Visual inspection method

B. Palpation method

A. Visual inspection method

- Service crate and animal

Procedure

- Secure the animal in a service crate in a comfortable standing position and observe the movements of the left paralumbar fossa at the left lateral abdominal region.
- Take note of how many ripples move in five minutes to determine the amount of rumen contractions.

B. Palpation method

- Service crate and animal.

Procedure

- Secure the animal in a service crate in a comfortable standing position.
- Then put your fist in the paralumbar fossa of the left flank, and press it, as illustrated in Fig.3.1. After some initial pressure, withdraw your fist and repress it in the same spot.

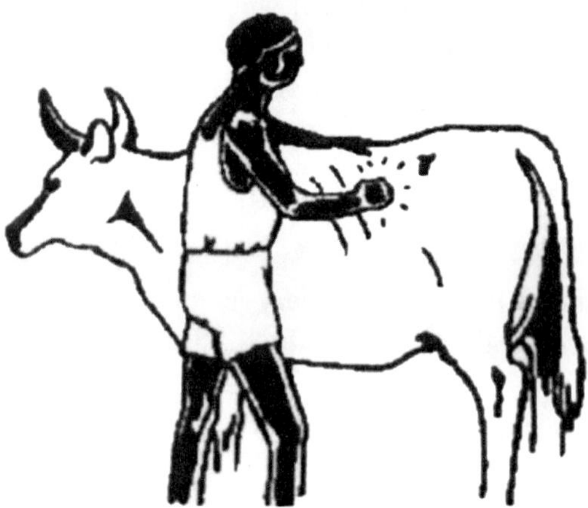

Fig. 3.1: Illustration of recording of rumen movements by palpation method.

- Count the rumen movements on your fist for 5 minutes. To confirm, do the same on the right side, which has no such contractions.
- Practice it in different animals under various conditions such as resting, feeding, rumination, etc.

Hypomotility

- Indigestion, traumatic reticuloperitonitis, rumen impaction, toxemia, dehydration, hypocalcaemia, etc.

Hypermotility

- Normally, coarse, fibrous feed stimulates the the greatest reticulorumen motility frequency and intensity.
- Pathological conditions like vagus indigestion, diaphragmatic hernia, early stage of bloat, etc.

3.2. Collection of Rumen Fluid

Rumen fluid (RF) is collected in order to perform ruminal fluid analysis. RF examination is crucial for determining the functional activity of the rumen, digestibility trials, and diagnosis of various disorders (rumen acidosis, for example) related to the fore stomach of ruminants. The digestibility of a nutrient is determined by performing digestibility trials on live animals. It is important for the evaluation of the nutritive value of feeds. Rumen microbial composition is influenced by diet, sampling, and handling practices. RF can be stored at ambient temperature for roughly 9 hours and refrigerated for 24 hours.

Method for collection of rumen fluid

A. By rumen fluid extraction pump.

B. Through rumen fistula.

C. By hypodermic needle.

D. Manual method from slaughtered animals.

3.2.a. By rumen fluid extraction pump

Materials required

- Ruminal fluid extraction pump: It consists of (a) specially designed suction strainer, (b) 4.0-meter-long nylon tube with perforations at the tip, (c) suction pump, and (d) an air-tight sampling container with a two-way “T” connection.
- Liquid paraffin, rumen collection bottle (500 mL), mouth gag, etc.

Procedure

- Secure the animal in a service crate with nose grips in a comfortable position.
- Open the mouth and then apply a mouth gag to keep the animal’s mouth open. Then gently pull out the tongue to one side.
- Apply liquid paraffin to the tube to facilitate passage.
- Insert the tube into the rumen through the mouth and esophagus. Some resistance is felt as it approaches the cardia, indicating that it has reached the ventral sac of the rumen.

Advantages

- Ethically acceptable.
- RF can be extracted from a live animal without the need for surgery.

Disadvantages

- Difficult procedure, and implicates a considerable stress to animals. It may also injury to esophagus.
- Saliva frequently contaminates RF samples.
- It is not possible to collect frequent and representative samples.

3.2.b. Through rumen fistula

It is an invasive procedure. A permanent fistula or cannula is fixed on the animal's left flank. The fistula is closed by a 25-125 mm cannula, a screw, a metal plate, or a hard rubber tube. Remove the screw and collect RF from 4-6 various locations in the rumen to obtain a representative sample of the entire rumen.

Materials required

- Fistulated or cannulated animals, 14-16 gauge sterilized needle, rumen collection bottle (500 mL), etc.

Procedure

- Press the skin over a hollow region of the left flank with one palm to bring it into contact with the rumen wall.
- Insert a 14-16 gauge sterile needle into the rumen by stabbing.
- Collect RF by inserting a syringe into the needle.

Advantages

- It is the simplest way for collecting RF from live animals.
- It is a reference method for collecting representative RF samples.

Disadvantages

- Ethical and practical issues, such as the necessity for surgical facilities.
- Require constant postoperative care to avoid infection.

- Reduce the economic value of the fistulated animals.
- Require long-term maintenance costs.

3.2.c. By hypodermic needle

Materials required

- Animal, hypodermic needle (6 inch), syringe, antiseptic, rumen collection bottle, etc.

Procedure

- Secure the animal in a service crate in a comfortable position.
- Clean and disinfect the lower part of the left flank.
- Insert the hypodermic needle into the rumen at the lower region of the left flank.
- Collect the RF sample with a syringe attached to the needle.

Advantages

- RF can be obtained from live animals.
- A standard procedure for collecting RF from young ruminants.

Disadvantage

- It is not feasible to collect a representative sample on a regular basis.

3.2.d. Manual method from slaughtered animals

- Thermic bottle (500 mL) filled with hot water (40°C), thermal bag or portable cooler box, thermometer, plastic beaker, colander or strainer, knife and spatula, gloves, gown, nylon socks, helmet, goggles, facemask, etc.

Procedure

- Collect about 200-300 g of rumen content by hand and squeeze it into the plastic beaker using a strainer or colander. Repeat this procedure until approximately 500 mL of RF is collected. Discard the hot water from a thermic bottle and fill it to the brim with the filtered RF; close immediately; no air should remain in the bottle.
- Put the RF-filled plastic beaker in the thermal bag then transport it immediately to the laboratory.

Advantages

- Ethically acceptable approach.
- Reduce stress and suffering in animals by eliminating an invasive RF collection procedure.

Disadvantage

- The time between the animal's death and the RF collection should be no more than 15 minutes.

3.3. Estimation of Total Volatile Fatty Acids (TVFA)

The main end products of microbial carbohydrate digestion in ruminants are VFAs, primarily acetic, propionic, and butyric acids. Protein fermentation produces small amounts of VFAs as well as short branched chain VFAs such as isoacid, isobutyric acid, and isovaleric acid. VFAs are absorbed through the rumen wall by (a) passive diffusion and (b) facilitate diffusion in exchange with bicarbonate.

In ruminant animals, VFAs are the primary source of energy for maintenance, growth, reproduction, and milk production. Acetate is the most abundant VFA in circulation, and it is used by the majority of body tissue to produce Acetyl-CoA, which is then used in the TCA cycle to produce ATP. It is also used in the production of long-chain fatty acids and is the primary precursor in the synthesis of body fat. Propionate is the only VFA used in the process of gluconeogenesis. Butyric acid is found in the general circulation as β-OH-butyrate. β-OH-butyrate is an energy source and a primary source of short to medium chain fatty acids.

Rumen fluid contains VFA. Hence, the TVFA can be estimated from the strained rumen liquor (SRL). When SRL is distilled in the presence of a scarisbrick's buffer, the VFAs are liberated and transformed into vapours. These vapours are condensed, distilled, and then titrated against alkali in the presence of an indicator to determine the amount of TVFA in the SRL.

Materials required

- Weighing balance, markham appartus, heating mantle, burette, conical flasks, pipette, wash bottle, ice, etc.
- Strained rumen liquor (rumen liquor is filtered with a muslin cloth to obtain SRL).

Reagents

1. Scarisbrick's buffer: It contains
   a. Potassium oxalate 10%: Dissolve 10 g of potassium oxalate in distilled water, and make the volume 100 mL with distilled water (solution-A).
   b. Oxalic acid (5 %): Dissolve 5 g of oxalic acid in distilled water, and make the volume 100 mL with distilled water (solution-B). Prepare freshly at the time of the experiment.
   c. Then mix the solution: A and solution-B.
2. 0.01 N NaOH.
3. Phenolphthalein indicator: Dissolve 0.1 g of phenolphthalein in 50 mL of ethanol and add to it 50 mL of distilled water.

Procedure

- Connect a round bottom flask with a volume of 2 litres to the Markham apparatus as illustrated in Fig. 3.2, and keep it on the heating mantle to allow the water to boil.
- Fill the inner jacket of the Markham apparatus with 1 mL of filtered rumen fluid and 1 mL of buffer.
- Put the stopper on. Then add a small amount of water to ensure airtightness.
- Allow the sample to boil on the heating mantle.
- Close the outlet of the outer jacket with the help of a pinch cork, once the water starts boiling.
- Collect about 50 mL of distillate in a conical flask, keeping the flask on the ice bath, as illustrated in Fig. 3.2.
- Add a few drops of phenolphthalein to the distillate, and titrate the distillate with 0.01N NaOH till the pink colour develops.
- Read the volume of 0.01 NaOH used for titration on the burette.
- Calculate the TVFA in the rumen liquor using the formula below. TVFA is expressed in mmol/L.

  TVFA in mmol rumen liquor = Volume of 0.01N NaOH used $\times 10$

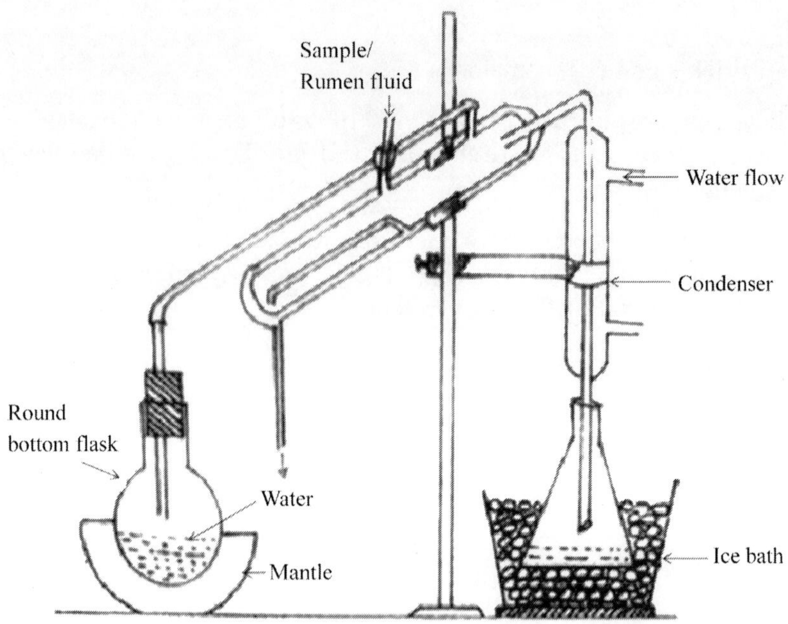

Fig. 3.2: Illustration of assemble markham's apparatus for the collection of distillate

Note

- In the rumen liquor, the concentration of TVFAs usually ranges from 70 to 150 mmol/L. The molar ratio of VFAs (acetic acid, propionic acid, and butyric acid) is around 70: 20: 10.
- The total concentration of VFAs varies greatly depending on the diet of the animal, the time of rumen liquor collection, the interval since the last meal, and the animals' overall health.
- Roughage (cellulose-rich diet) and grain (amylase-rich diet) diets undergo microbial fermentation, which results in the production of VFAs (acetic, propionic, and butyric acids) in the ratios of 75:15:10 and 70:25:05, respectively.

Table 3.1: Reference value of volatile fatty acids (VFAs) in the rumen liquor of cattle and sheep fed on various diets.

Sl No	Animals	Diets	Total VFAs (mmol/ L)	Individual VFA (molar proportions)			
				Acetic	Propionic	Butyric	Others
1	Sheep	Young ryegrass herbage	107	0.60	0.24	0.12	0.04
2	Cattle	Mature ryegrass herbage	137	0.64	0.22	0.11	0.03
3	Cattle	Grass silage	108	0.74	0.17	0.07	0.03
4	Sheep	Chopped Lucerne hay	113	0.63	0.23	0.10	0.04
		Ground Lucerne hay	105	0.65	0.19	0.11	0.05
5	Cattle	Long hay (0.4) and Concentrate (0.6)	96	0.61	0.18	0.13	0.08
		Pelleted Hay (0.4) and Concentrates (0.6)	140	0.50	0.30	0.11	0.09
6	Sheep	Hay :concentrate					
		1.0: 0.0	97	0.66	0.22	0.09	0.03
		0.8 : 0.2	80	0.61	0.25	0.11	0.03
		0.6: 0.4	87	0.61	0.23	0.13	0.02
		0.4 : 0.6	76	0.52	0.34	0.12	0.03
		0.2 : 0.8	70	0.40	0.40	0.15	0.05
7	Cattle	Barley (no ciliate protozoa in rumen)	146	0.48	0.28	0.14	0.10
8	Cattle	Barley (ciliate protozoa present in rumen)	105	0.62	0.14	0.18	0.06

Table 3.2: Mineral concentrations of ruminal fluid in relation to better cellulolysis:

Sl.No.	Minerals	Mineral concentration
1.	Potassium	0.05 – 0.26 g/ L
2.	Calcium	20-40 mg/L
3.	Phosphorus	283- 1033 mg/ L
4.	Magnesium	1-25 mg/L
5.	Sodium	0.04 -0.2 g/L
6.	Iron	0.5-12.5 mg/L
7.	Zinc	7.5 mg/L
8.	Manganese	7.5 mg/L
9.	Molybdenum	0.07-0.14 mg/L

3.4 Estimation of Ammonia-Nitrogen

Ruminant animals' diets contain proteins, which are digested by rumen microbes into peptides and amino acids. Further, some amino acids are converted into organic acids, ammonia, and carbon dioxide during the degradation process. Hence, strained rumen liquor (SRL) is used to estimate total ammonia-nitrogen.

When SRL is treated with potassium carbonate, ammonia is released, which is absorbed by boric acid and used to titrate against standard sulfuric acid to estimate the ammonia nitrogen concentration.

Materials required

- Conway diffusion disc (it has two chambers: an outer chamber and an inner chamber), pipette, burette and strained rumen liquor.

Reagents

- Boric acid (2 %) solution.
- Mix methyl red indicator (dissolve 66 mg of methyl red, and 33 mg of methylene blue or bromocresol green in 100 mL of alcohol).
- Boric acid solution (1 mL of mixed indicator in 100 mL of 2 % boric acid, and mix it).
- 0.01 N sulfuric acid (H_2SO_4).
- Potassium carbonate.

Procedure

- Add 2 mL of 2% boric acid solution with an indicator into the conway diffusion disc's inner chamber.

- Add 1 mL of SRL and 1 mL of a saturated solution of potassium carbonate opposite to SRL in the outer chamber of the disc in such a manner that SRL and potassium carbonate are not mixed.
- Put the cover on the disc and fix it properly to make it airtight.
- Gently tilt and rotate the disc to mix the SRL and potassium carbonate in the outer chamber.
- Leave the disc for an hour at a temperature between 37 °C to 38 °C in the oven. The boric acid will turn green after ammonia absorption.
- Titrate the contents of the inner chamber against 0.01N sulfuric acid to the endpoint (colour changes to violet, i.e., original colour), using a fine-tip burette, and note the amount of H_2SO_4 used.
- Calculate the total ammonia-nitrogen in the rumen liquor using the formula below.

$$NH_3\text{-N mg/dL of SRL} = \text{Volume of 0.01 N } H_2SO_4 \text{ used} \times 14.$$

Note

- The reference range for ammonia-nitrogen in large ruminants (cattle and buffalo) is between 6 and 15 mg/dL. Animal hosts become poisonous when ammonia-nitrogen concentrations exceed 80 mg/dL.
- The amount of total ammonia-nitrogen in the rumen liquors fluctuates significantly depending on the animal's health, the time of rumen liquor collection, and diets higher in NPN compounds such as urea or feed treated with NPN.

3.5. Bacteria and Protozoa Count

Rumen microorganisms are crucial for the development of the digestive tract in newborns or nursing calves. They also profoundly influence the host's physiological and immune systems. The rumen microbes are not present at birth. These microorganisms multiply depending on the kinds of feed supplied to calves and their age as they grow. The rumen is fully developed and has an adult microbial population at about 9 weeks of age.

The rumen contains a variety of microbes, which include bacteria (10^{10}-10^{11} cells/mL), protozoa (10^4-10^6/mL), fungi (10^3-10^5/mL), bacteriophages (10^8-10^9/mL), yeast, etc. In the rumen, there are about 7000 different bacterial species. These microbes secrete digestive enzymes such as cellulases, hemicellulases, pectinlyases, fructosanses, proteases, peptidases, amylases, etc that enable microbial digestion in the rumen.

Rumen protozoa are commonly detected in ruminant animals' high-grain diets. Although protozoa are not directly involved in the digestion of proteins and carbohydrates, they are essential for bypassing polyunsaturated- fatty acids (PUFAs), proteins, and small amounts of unfermented starch, from the rumen to the lower gastrointestinal tract.

Rumen fungus make up between 5 and 10% of the entire rumen microbiota at any given moment. Fungi aid in the hydrolysis of certain ester bonds between lignin, hemicelluloses or cellulose, etc.

Methods of counting rumen bacteria and protozoa

- Direct counts or viable counts: A direct counting method is used to determine the overall number of bacteria or protozoa, with little differentiation between the numerous species that make up those groupings of organisms.
- Using Neubauer's counting chamber.
- Colorimetric and spectrophotometric methods.

Among them, employing Neubauer's counting chamber to count bacteria and protozoa is more convenient.

Materials required

- Strained rumen liquor (SRL), haemocytometer, microscope, pipette, coverslip, and muslin cloth.

Reagents

- Gentian violet crystals and formaldehyde.

Procedure

- Collect rumen liquor and filter it with a muslin cloth to obtain SRL.
- Add a few drops of formaldehyde solution to the SRL to kill the microbes. Then, add a few crystals of gentian violet to give the microbes a recognizable stain.
- Charge the Neubauer's counting chamber after adding a drop of fluid (the reaction mixture of SRL, formaldehyde, and stain) through the pipette's tip.

- Focus the Neubauer's counting chamber under a high power objective (40x) of the microscope to count the number of microorganisms in five medium squares, as RBC counting.
- Count the bacteria and protozoa, separately.

Calculation

The volume of 5 medium squares used for microbial count is 1/50 cu mm (mm^3). As a result, multiply the number of bacteria or protozoa by 50,000. (50×1000). The total number of microorganisms is expressed in terms of per mL of rumen fluid.

Note

- Rumen microenvironment conditions, including pH, are extremely sensitive to rumen microbes. Because they are strict anaerobes, bacteria can't survive in an oxygen-rich environment.
- Rumen microorganisms can be affected by a variety of factors, including diet, genetics, environment, and an animal's overall health.

Table 3.3: List of common microbes found in the rumen:

Grouping of microbes based on types of substratefermented	**Species**
Cellulose degrading bacteria	*Fibrobacter succinogenes (Bacteroides succinogenes)*
	Ruminococcus flavefaciens
	Ruminococcus albus
	Clostridium cellobioparum
	Clostridium longisporum
	Clostridium lochheadii
	Eubacterium cellulosolvens (Cillobacterium cellulosolvens)
Hemicellulose degradingbacteria	*Butyrivibrio fibrisolvens*
	Prevotella ruminicola (Bacteroides ruminicola)
	Eubacterium xylanophilum
	Euniformis
	Ruminococcus species
Starch degrading bacteria	*Streptococcus bovis*
	Ruminobacter amylophilus (*Bacteroides amylophilu*)
	Prevetella ruminicola (*Bacteroides ruminicola*)
	Succinimonas amylolytica

Grouping of microbes based on types of substratefermented	Species
Sugars/dextrin's degrading bacteria	*Succinivibrio dextrinosolvens*
	Succinivibrio amylolytica
	Selenomonas ruminantium
	Lactobacillus acidophilus
	L casei
	L fermentum
	L plantarum
	L brevis

Grouping of microbes based on types of substrate fermented	Species
	L helveticus
	L vituinus
	L ruminis
	Treponema bryanta
	Bifidobacterium globosum,
	B longum
	B thermophilum
	B ruminale
	B ruminantium
Pectin-degrading bacteria	*Treponema saccharophilum*
	Lachnospira multiparus
	Butyrivibrio fibrisolvens
	Bacteroides ruminicola
	Lachnospira multiparus
	Succinivibrio dextrinosolvens
	Treponema bryantii
	Streptococcus bovis
Protein degrading bacteria	*Prevotella ruminicola*
	Bacteroides amylophilus
	B ruminicola
	Butyrivibrio fibrisolvens
	Streptococcus bovis
	Ruminobacter amylophilus
	Clostridium bifermentans

Grouping of microbes based on types of substrate fermented	Species
Lipolytic bacteria	*Anaerovibrio lipolytica*
	Butyrivibrio fibrisolvens
	Treponema bryantii
	Eubacterium species
	Fusocillus species
	Micrococcus species
Lactate-degrading bacteria	*Selenomonas lactilytica*
	Megasphaera elsdeni
Methanogenic bacteria	*Methanobrevibacter ruminantium*
	M formicium
	M mobile
Lactic acid-utilizing bacteria	*Megasphaera elsdenii*
	Selenomonas ruminantium
Urea-utilizing bacteria	*Succinivibrio dextrinosolvens*
	Succinivibrio species
	Bacteroides ruminicola
	Ruminococcus bromii
	Butyrivibrio species
	Treponema bryantii

3.6. Digestive Action of Amylase on Starch

Carbohydrates are the main source of energy. Starch is the most prevalent carbohydrate in the diet. Starch is a polysaccharide that contains amylose and amylopectin. Amylose is made up of multiple glucose monomers linked together linearly by α-1-4-glycosidic linkages. Amylopectin is a monomer of branched glucose. Starch is hydrolyzed by α-amylase. The overall reaction is as follows:

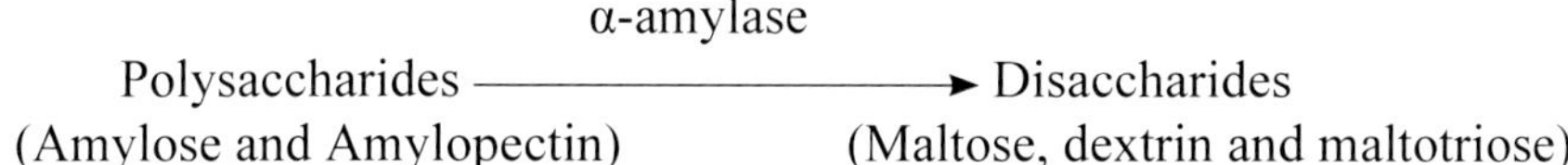

Salivary α-amylase is present in the saliva of humans, pigs, and some birds.

1. Collection of saliva

The collection of the animal's saliva necessitates skill. There are several methods for collecting pig saliva, which are as follows:

(a) Traditional rope-chew method

- Hang a rope of approximately 5-15 mm thick in such a way that it reaches the pig's shoulders.
- Allow the pig to chew on it for 15-45 minutes.
- Then collect the fluids from the ropes in a sterile plastic bag.

(b) Cable lock-assisted swab method

- Tie a swab at one end of a cable lock and serve it to a mature pig.
- Allow the pig to chew on it for 2 minutes to achieve optimal oral fluid absorption.
- Thereafter, take out the swab carefully from the cable knot and place it in a collection tube to collect saliva samples after spinning at 10,000 rpm for 5 minutes (4°C).
- Store the collected saliva at −80°C for subsequent biochemical analysis.

(c) Rope-assisted swab method

- Wrap the swab with a clip over the buccal cavity and behind the ears, making sure to place the swab in the centre of the buccal cavity. The swab is tied with nylon thread in the middle of an undyed cotton rope.
- Allow the pig to chew on it for 2 minutes to ensure sufficient absorption of the oral fluids.
- After that, carefully take out the swab and place it in a collection tube for collecting saliva samples after centrifugation at 10,000 rpm for 5 minutes (4°C).
- Store the collected saliva at -80°C for subsequent biochemical analysis.

2. Test for the presence of maltose in saliva

Materials required

- Test tube, beaker, water bath, and marker.

Reagents and sample

- 1% Starch solution, Benedict's solution, and saliva.

Procedure

- Take four test tubes and mark them one to four.

- Add starch, saliva, HCI and distilled water to all marked test tubes as follows:

  Test tube-1: 3 mL of 1% starch solution and 3 mL of distilled water.

  Test tube-2: 3 mL of 1% starch solution and 3 mL of saliva.

  Test tube-3: 3 mL 1% of starch solution, 3 mL of saliva and 5 drops of conc. HCI.

  Test tube-4: 3 mL1% of starch solution, 3 mL of distilled water and drops of conc. HCI.

- Incubate all tubes for 1 hour at 37^0C.
- After incubation, pour half of the reaction mixture from each test tube into the newly marked test tubes.
- Add 4 mL of benedict's solution in each tube and incubate all test tubes in boiling water for 4 minutes.
- Observe how the colour changes. The transformation of the reaction colour to green, brown, orange, or red indicates the hydrolysis of starch into maltose. If there is no change in colour, starch has not been digested.

3.7. Digestive Action of Pepsin on Proteins *in-vitro*

The behaviour of the food matrix in the acidic conditions of the stomach of animals and humans can influence the dynamic of gastric emptying and the postprandial appearance of amino acids in the blood. As a result, the gastric phase of digestion is critical to the kinetics of protein digestion and absorption. Pepsin is a digestive enzyme that is released by the stomach's cells. In the stomach, pepsinogen is converted to pepsin at pH 2-3.5. Pepsin activity is highly sensitive to pH.

$$\text{Cupric ion } (Cu^{2+}) + \text{reducing sugar} \xrightarrow[\text{Heat}]{\text{Alkali}} \text{Cuprous ions} + \text{Oxidized sugar}$$

Materials required

- Test tubes, pipettes, and water bath.

Reagents and sample

- Casein, egg albumin, fibrin or milk, 5 % HCI, NaOH and 5 % pepsin.

Procedure

- Take four test tubes and mark them one to four.
- Take equal amounts of fresh egg albumin or fibrin in four test tubes, numbered from one to four.
- Add pepsin, HCl, water, and NaOH in all test tubes as follows- Test tube no: 1 Add 3 mL of pepsin + 3 mL of HCI
- Test tube no: 2 Add 3 mL of pepsin + 3 mL of water Test tube no: 3 Add 3 mL of water + 3 mL of HCI Test tube no: 4 Add 3 mL of pepsin + 3 mL of NaOH.
- Incubate all test tubes in a water bath at 37°C for 30 minutes.
- Take note of how many eggs were broken. They are graded as (+++) entirely digested, (++) moderately digested, (+) slightly digested, and (-) no change.

3.8. Digestive Action of Trypsin on Proteins

Trypsin is a digestive enzyme secreted by the pancreas. It is an endopeptidase enzyme that serves two main functions: (a) protein digestion and (b) activation of all inactive digestive enzymes (zymogens) secreted by the pancreas, as shown below.

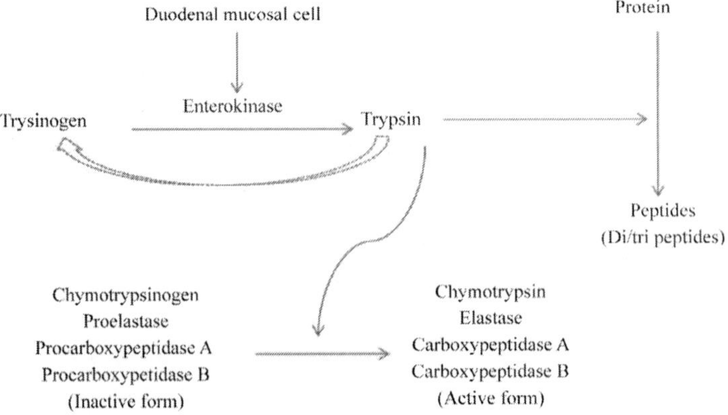

When casein, egg albumin, or fibrin solutions are treated with trypsin solution, they hydrolyze into peptides. The end products are examined *in vitro* to evaluate how trypsin digests proteins.

Materials required

- Test tubes, pipettes, sprit lamp and water bath.

Reagents

- Trypsin solution (1%): Dissolve 1g of trypsin powder in 100 mL of 2% Na_2CO_3.
- Casein solution (1%) prepare in normal saline.
- Ninhydrin solution (1%) prepare in ethanol.
- Trichloroacetic acid (5%) prepare in distilled water.

Procedure

- Take two test tubes and mark them as "C" (control) and "T" (test).
- Add 2.0 mL of casein solution to both tubes in addition to 2.0 mL of trypsin solution in 'T' and 2.0 mL of distilled water in 'C' and mix them separately.
- Incubate both tubes at 37^0C in a water bath for 30 minutes.
- After incubation, take out the tubes and perform the following tests to determine the presence of protein in the reaction mixture:

Ninhydrin test

- Take a portion of each tube in other labelled tubes as "T" and "C". Then, add a few drops (0.1 mL) of Ninhydrin solution and heat the tubes until they boil over a spirit lamp.
- Cool the tubes and observe the change in colour of the solution. Ninhydrin gives a blue-purple or brown colour with proteins, peptides, peptones, and amino acids; the colour is more intense with hydrolyzed proteins.

Precipitation test

- To the remaining portion of both tubes, add 0.5 mL of trichloroacetic acid solution and observe the appearance of precipitates.
- Trichloroacetic acid precipitates intact proteins while leaving hydrolyzed products in a transparent solution.

Note

Digestive enzymes are released throughout the digestive tract that aid in the chemical reaction or breakdown of ingested large nutrient macromolecules into simpler molecules simpler molecules for utilization by an organism. Enzymatic activity is required for normal growth, reproduction, and metabolism.

4

Respiration and Spirometry

4.0. Introduction

The main function of the respiratory system is to exchange O_2 and CO_2 between the atmosphere, blood, and cells, which are necessary for animal survival. The circulatory and respiratory systems work together to provide oxygen to cells while eliminating CO_2. O_2 consumption and CO_2 production are determined by cell metabolic activity.

Respiratory volumes or lung volumes refer to the volumes of gas in the lungs at any given point during the respiratory cycle. These volumes vary according to the animals' physiological state, ambient factors, and health status. This is why; measurements of lung volumes are helpful in understanding the pathophysiology of the respiratory system.

4.1. Recording of Respiration and Spirometry

Spirometry is a valuable method for assessing lung pathophysiology. It is frequently used in pulmonary function tests (PFTs), especially in humans. In this test, a device known as '**spirometer**' is used to measure the volume and speed of air that an individual can inhale and exhale. Spirometry is possibly the simplest of PFTs. PFTs can help the clinician define the abnormalities in the respiratory system and understand the pathophysiology of the lungs.

Spirometry is the gold standard method for diagnosing obstructive respiratory diseases in humans. This method has also shown promise in veterinary medicine, particularly for monitoring airway pressures, flows, and volumes during small animal and equine anaesthesia.

Most spirometers display a graph called a spirogram. Spirometry provides lung volumes such as tidal volume, inspiratory reserve volume, and expiratory reserve volume. Inspiratory reserve volume and expiratory reserve volume can be used to detect, characterize, and quantify the severity of lung diseases.

Materials required

- Airtight face mask and spirometer.

Spirometer consists (Fig 4.1) of:

(a) A drum inverted over a water chamber.

(b) A weight counterbalancing the drum.

(c) An oxygen cylinder.

(d) A rubber tube that connects the mouth with a gas chamber.

(e) A recording drum.

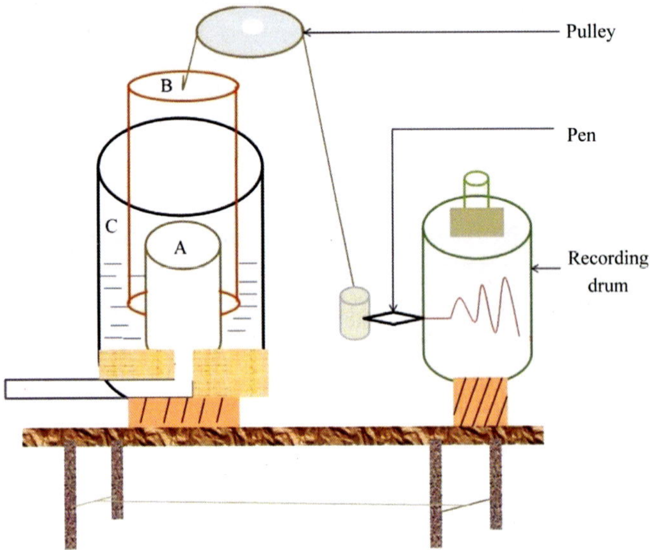

Fig. 4.1: Spirometer (water-seal type)

Procedure

- Secure the animal in a comfortable position.
- Tie the airtight face mask around an awake animal's mouth and nostrils.
- Then, connect an airtight face mask to a spirometer.
- Set the spirometer to zero and then let the animal to breathe in and out in a calm state (normal quiet respiration).
- Take note of the volume of air. This amount of air is known as tidal volume.
- Then allow the animal to inhale maximally, followed by maximal exhalation, to record vital capacity. However, the animals' cooperation is required. For example, in order to record the inspiratory reserve

volume and the forced expiratory volume in animals, the test subject must forcefully expel air following a large inhalation.

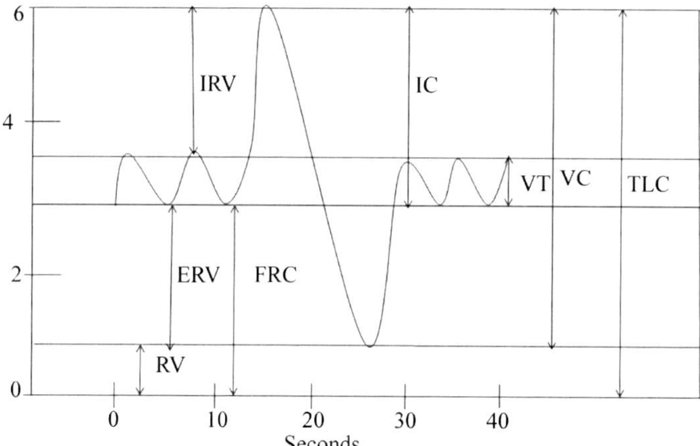

Fig. 4.2: Illustration of lung volumes and capacities based on a volume-time spirogram

- Lung volumes are TV= Tidal Volume, IRV= Inspiratory Reserve Volume, ERV= Expiratory Reserve Volume, and RV= Residual Volume.
- Lung capacities are IC = Inspiratory Capacity, VC=Vital Capacity, FVC= Force Vital Capacity, and TLC = Total Lung Capacity.

Table 4.1: Explanation of common test values in spirometry:

Abbreviation	Name	Description
TV	Tidal Volume	The amount of air inhaled or exhaled during a single breath without forced conditions.
IC	Inspiratory capacity	The volume of air that can be inspired after normal expiration. $IC = V_T + IRV$
IRV	Inspiratory Reserve Volume	The maximum additional air that can be inhaled at the end of a normal inspiration. $IRV=IC-V_T$
ERV	Expiratory Reserve Volume	Refers to the maximum volume of air that can be exhaled at the end of a normal expiration.
VC	Vital capacity	Refers to the maximum amount of air that can be inhaled after maximum amount has been exhaled. $VC=V_T+IRV+ERV$ or $VC= IC+ERV$
RV	Residual volume	Refers to the amount of air remains in the lungs after forceful expiration.

Abbreviation	Name	Description
FVC	Forced VitalCapacity	The volume of air that can be exhaled out by an animal at maximal speed and effort after full inspiration.
TLC	Total Lung Capacity	Maximum volume of air present in the lungs. or Vital Capacity plus Residual Volume. Or the sum of all volume compartments.
FEV_1	Forced Expiratory Volume in 1 second	Represents the maximum volume of air that can beexhaled in a forced way in the first second after taking a deep breath.
FEV_1/ FVC	FEV_1 %	This is the ratio of FEV_1 to FVC.
FIVC	Forced Inspiratory Vital Capacity	The maximum air volume that can be inhaled.
PIF	Peak InspiratoryFlow	The forced maximum flow that can be achieved during inhalation.
PEF	Peak Expiratory Flow	The maximum airflow that can be forced during exhalation.
MVV	Maximum Voluntary Ventilation	A measure of the maximum amount of air that can be inhaled and exhaled in one minute and is measured in liters per minute.

Note: Measurement of absolute lung volume, RV, FRC, and TLC are technically more challenging in domestic animals.

Tidal volume and respiratory frequency

The Table 4.2 below displays the average tidal volume and reference value for the respiratory frequency of domestic animals.

Table 4.2: Average tidal volume and respiratory frequency for several domestic animals:

Sl. No	Animal	Average body weight (kg)	Conditions	Respiratory frequency (breaths/ min)	Tidal volume (mL/kg)
1	Holstein cow Jersey cow	516 405	Standing Standing	26 27	8.20, S. D. 1.29 8.44, S.D. 1.40
2	Horse (Thoroughbred)	486	Resting	10	15.4, S. D. 0.76
3	Dog (Beagles)	13.8	Pentobarbital anesthesia	23	15.7, S. D. 5.8
4	Cat	3.7	Pentobarbital anesthesia	30	9.2

S.D.: Standard deviation.

Interpretation of spirometry results

Interpretation	FVC	FEV1	FEV1/FVC%
Normal spirometry	Normal	Normal	Normal
Airway obstruction	Low or normal	Low	Low
Lung restriction	Low	Low	Normal
Combination of obstruction and restriction	Low	Low	Low

Factors influence respiratory frequency

The reference interval of respiratory frequency varies from species to species in animals. A physiological rise in respiratory frequency is evident after extensive activities or work, fear, anger, sexual excitement or restlessness, anxiety or tension, and stress, advanced pregnancy, young animals, etc.

Increased respiratory frequency is also seen in animals confined in a poorly ventilated room during very cold or hot weather, with a degree of filling of the digestive tract, an obese body condition, as well as pathological conditions or states of health such as fever, pleurisy, peritonitis, pneumonia, pneumothorax, the massive collapse of the lungs, edema of the upper respiratory tract, anemic conditions, cardiac disorders, partial obstruction of the respiratory passages, etc.

The following technical terms are useful for describing the state of the breathing pattern:

- Eupnea: It is the state of normal, quiet breathing with the usual respiratory rate of an individual animal.
- Apnea: It is the state of transient cessation of breathing or absence of respiration.
- Dyspnea: It is the state of difficult or labored breathing.
- Tachypnea: It is the state of excessive rapidity of breathing.
- Bradypnea: It is the state of abnormal slowness of breathing.
- Hyperpnea: It is the state of breathing in which frequency, depth, or both are increased.
- Hypopnea: It is the state of breathing in which frequency, depth, or both are decreased.
- Polypnea: It is the state of the quick, shallow, panting kind of respiration.
- Pneumonia: It is an inflammation of the lungs.

- Atelectasis: It is the state of failure of the alveoli to open or remain open. It usually includes one or more relatively small portions of the lung. The most prevalent reasons are full obstruction of the airway and a lack of surfactant in the fluids lining the alveoli.

5

Excretory System: Comprehensive Insights into Urine Analysis

5.0. Introduction

The kidneys play a vital role in maintaining water and electrolyte balance (such as chloride, potassium, calcium, hydrogen, magnesium, and phosphate ions). It also regulates the acid-base balance of the blood, arterial blood pressure, and osmotic pressure of the body.

Urine is an excretory body fluid, and it consists of water and water-soluble waste products, which are removed from the bloodstream by the kidneys and excreted as urine. Normally, the kidneys receive about 22% of the cardiac output. According to Arthur Cushny (1866-1926), there are three steps involved in urine formation in the nephrons: glomerular filtration, tubular reabsorption, and tubular secretion. When the kidneys are injured, their regulatory activities are disrupted, resulting in a change in the quality and quantity of urine. Urine is composed of the following components:

Normal urine constituents	Abnormal urine constituents
Water (about 95% of urine)	Glucose
Urea	Proteins
Creatinine	Bile pigments
Uric acids	Blood cells
Electrolytes	Cast and microbes

This is the reason why a urine analysis is a common test to evaluate the pathophysiology of the urinary system in general and the kidneys in particular, as well as to aid in the differential diagnosis of certain diseases.

5.1. Collection of Urine

The urine specimen must be collected properly to make a reliable urinalysis. Improper collection may invalidate the results of the laboratory procedures, no matter how carefully and skillfully the tests are performed.

Methods of urine collection

In animals, a urine sample is normally collected in a sterile specimen container when it is voided or excreted voluntarily. This type of urine sample is called a "free-catch" sample. The other methods are:

a. Manual method using polythene bags

b. By catheterization

5.1.a. Manual Method Using Polythene Bags

This approach is used for quantitative examination of a urine sample. In cows, buffaloes, sheep, and goats, one can stimulate the urethra through the vulva, which allows the animal to urinate. Urine samples from large animals can also be collected by applying pressure to the urinary bladder through the rectum.

Materials required

- Polythene bags, rope, sterile container, etc.

Procedure

- Tie a polythene bag across the urethra with a rope around the back of large animals.
- Collect the polythene bag once it has been filled with urine or at different time intervals.
- Then transfer the urine sample from the polythene bag into a sterile container and label it.

5.1.b. By Catheterization

Catheterization is the preferred method for the collection of urine samples for bacterial culture and sensitivity tests.

Materials required

- Catheter, vaginal speculum, sterile syringe, antiseptic solution, sterile container, etc.

Procedure

- Clean the genitalia with soapy water and apply antiseptic solutions.
- Gently insert the catheter into the bladder through the urethra after dilating the vagina with the vaginal speculum. The urinary orifice is located slightly below the clitoris and 10cm inside the lower commissure

of the valve in cows, sheep, and goats. If an obstruction is felt while inserting the catheter, do not apply too much pressure.

- After that, connect a sterile syringe to the catheter and draw urine from the bladder into the syringe.
- Then, transfer the urine sample from the syringe into a sterile container and label it.

Note: As specimen containers, use dark glass containers. Sunlight degrades bilirubin and urobilinogen in less than an hour. Also, the first portion of urine should be discarded, since it contains cellular debris, cells, and exudates drained from the urethra, prepuce, and genitals.

Sources of Errors in the Collection of Urine

- Use of an insufficient or incorrect amount of preservative.
- Partial loss of specimens or inclusion of two-morning specimens in the 24-hour collection.
- Inadequate mixing of the samples prior to urine analysis or examination.

5.2. Preservation of Urine Samples

The urine sample should be examined immediately after collection because some urine components are unstable. When a delay is anticipated, it must be kept at refrigerator temperature (4°C) without any preservatives. Because prolonged storage of urine at room temperature promotes bacterial growth, the breakdown of urea to ammonia, an increase in pH, precipitation of calcium and phosphates, oxidation of urobilinogen to urobilin, bacterial destruction of glucose, hemolysis, and cast formation.

Method of Preservation

A. Physical Methods

(a) Refrigeration

(b) Freezing

B. Chemical Method

The urine sample can be kept for a long period if the following chemical preservatives are used.

1. *Toluene*: To preserve the urine sample, add a layer of toluene over it. It is an antibacterial agent that can keep the urine sample safe for 24 hours.

2. *Formalin*: One drop of 40% formalin is adequate for 30 mL of urine.
3. *Thymol*: It acts as an antimicrobial agent. 5-10 mL of 10 % thymol can preserve urine samples for up to 24 hours.
4. *Phenol*: Use one drop of phenol per 10 mL of urine to preserve it without significant deterioration.
5. *Chloroform*: It acts as an antimicrobial agent. The total amount of urine that an animal excretes in a day can be preserved with 5 mL of chloroform.
6. *Boric acid*: 1 g of boric acid is sufficient to preserve a urine sample taken over the course of a day.

Table 5.1: Methods of Preservation, and Their Advantages and Disadvantages:

Methods	Advantages	Disadvantages
Refrigeration	No chemical interference.	Only use for short period of time.
Freezing	For specimen transport.	May destroy formed elements.
Toluene	Preserves acetone, protein and reducing substance such as glucose, fructose, etc.	Inflammable.
Thymol	Preserve the most constituents of urine specimen.	May give a false reaction for albumin content.
Chloroform	Preserve urine aldosterone level.	Settles at the bottom of theurine containers.
Formaldehyde	Preserves formed elementsPrevents bacterial growth.	May interfere with sugar examination.
Boric acid	Preserves chemicals and formed elements.	Precipitate uric acid.

5.3. Methods of Urine Examination

Urine analysis can be classified into three types, which are as follows:

1. Physical examination
2. Chemical analysis
3. Microscopic examination

5.4 Physical Examination of Urine

The physical examination of the urine sample gives a hint for the subsequent urinalysis. This includes volume, colour, odour, transmittancy (appearance), pH, foam, and specific gravity.

5.4.1.a. Volume

The volume of urine excreted each day depends on age, size, and species of animals. It also depends on individual fluid intake, body temperature, climate, and health status. The reference value for urine void per day in domestic animals is shown in Table 5.2 below.

Table 5.2: Reference intervals for urine voided in domestic animals:

	Cattle	**Sheep**	**Goat**	**Horse**	**Dog**
Urine (Liters/day)	7-10	1-1.5	1-1.5	5-10	0.5-1.5

Procedure

- Collect urine voided within 24 hours by the animals or patients in urine specimen containers. Use a brown or dark-coloured specimen container to avoid direct sunlight contact with the collected urine sample and the interaction of sunlight with the chemicals.
- Measure the total amount of urine void using a graduated measuring cylinder.
- Calculate the amount in milliliters every 24 hours.

Abnormally higher amounts (polyuria), very low amounts (oliguria), and total cessation of urine excretion (anuria) are associated with some pathophysiological conditions in animals.

- *Polyuria*: Excess water intake, low protein diets, pregnancy, etc.
- *Oliguria:* Low water intake, during summer months, profuse sweating, high fever, high protein diet, dehydration, etc.
- *Anuria:* Cardiac failure, surgical shock, acute renal failure, etc.

5.4.1.b. Colour

Normal urine colour is derived from bilirubin, which is excreted into the intestine and is reabsorbed into the portal circulation as urobilinogen. Urobilin is the partially oxidized urobilinogen that is responsible for the yellow colour of urine.

Procedure

- Observe the colour of freshly voided urine samples in a test tube or a urinometer cylinder within 30 minutes of collection. If the colour of the urine sample is not documented within 30 minutes after collection, chemical changes occur, resulting in an incorrect result.

The aberrant colour of urine in animals varies depending on the contents of the urine sample. The colour of urine and conditions related with it are shown in Table-5.3 below.

Table 5.3: Urine colour and its associated conditions:

S.No	Colour of urine	Condition
1.	Pale yellow	Excess ingestion of water and pathological conditions such as pyometra, chronic interstitial nephritis, diabetes insipidus, etc.
2.	Brownish yellow	Dehydration, vomiting, diarrhoea, fever, insufficient water intake, etc.
3.	Brown	Jaundice or icterus. In horse, brown to black colour urine may be observed in a normal animal.
4.	Red	Presence of free haemoglobin or blood in the urine.
5.	Pus	Pyogenic infections of the kidney.
6.	Green	Medication with Methylene blue or Diazan
7.	Brown/coffee coloured	Haemoglobinuria or Myoglobinuria

5.4.1.c. Odour

Animals in good health usually have uremic urine because they have volatile acids in their freshly voided urine.

Procedure

- Take note of the smell or odour of a freshly urinated urine sample. The test result is based on how the technician interprets it.

Abnormal urine odour may result from aging of urine, disease (e.g., sweetish odour in diabetes mellitus, acetone odour in ketonuria) and diet. The bacterial breakdown of urea results in an ammonia-like urine odour. Some male species have a pungent odour in their urine. In general, the odour of the urine is not a diagnostic aid.

5.4.1.d. pH

The litmus paper technique is a simple and routinely used to determine the pH of a given urine sample. In this technique, pH of the urine sample is measured with either blue or red litmus paper.

Procedure

- Tear a piece of litmus paper.
- Then, dip the litmus paper into the freshly voided, well-mixed urine sample, and take it out immediately.

- Observe the blue litmus paper for any colour changes, and then compare them with the standard pH indicator. The acidity of the urine is indicated by the litmus paper turning from blue to red.

Reference value for urine pH

Urine pH fluctuates according to age, diet type, body metabolism, and species (Table 5.4). Additionally, it changes according to the animal's health, body temperature, climate, and fluid intake.

Table 5.4: Reference intervals for urine pH in various domestic animals:

Animals	Cattle	Sheep	Pig	Horse	Dog	Cat
pH	7.4-8.0	4.8 -7.5	Acidic or alkaline	8.0	6.0 -7.0	6.0-7.0

Acidic urine

- Normal in carnivores, calves, and foal, a diet with high protein, starvation, fever, acidosis (metabolic and respiratory), diabetes mellitus, uremia, diarrhea, dehydration, high muscular activity, etc.

Alkaline urine

- Normal in the case of herbivorous animals, vegetable diet, cystitis, urine retention, vomiting and alkaline therapy with sodium carbonate. Urinary tract obstruction, pyloric obstruction, salicylate intoxication, renal tubular acidosis, chronic renal failure, a respiratory disease that involves hyperventilation (blowing off carbon dioxide and development of alkalosis), etc.

5.4.1.e. Transmittancy

The transmittancy (appearance) of a freshly urinated urine sample can be checked by putting it up to the light in a test tube. The common terms used to describe the transmittancy of urine samples include clear, hazy, cloudy, very cloudy, and turbid. Normally, the urine should be transparent and clear.

- Clear urine: Freshly voided urine from healthy animals is usually clear.
- Cloudy urine: It may be pathological. A cloudy appearance could be caused by the presence of many epithelial cells, leucocytes, bacteria, calcium carbonate that looks like crystals, and mucus, as in the case of horses.
- Brown smoky urine: The urine contains pus and haematin.

5.4.1. f. Foam

A small amount of white foam may be produced by freshly urinated urine. Under specific abnormal physiological and metabolic conditions, the amount of foam may alter. For instance, the quantity of yellowish foam increases when the urine contains a lot of bile pigment. However, it cannot be used as a confirmation test for bilirubin in urine. Albuminuria is frequently accompanied by foam.

5.4.1.g. Specific Gravity

Specific gravity is the weight of a specific amount of solution relative to that of a similar volume of water at a particular temperature, usually 15°C. The concentration of dissolved solids influences the specific gravity of 24-hour urine samples.

Methods of measuring the specific gravity

A. Urinometer

B. Refractometer

A. Urinometer

The urinometer is a glass float with a graded stem on top that is weighted with mercury and has an air bulb above it (Fig. 5.1). A mercury scale is used to measure the weight. The range of the scale is 1.000 to 1.060.

Procedure

- Fill ¾th of the urinometer cylinder with urine.
- Place the urinometer in the urine-containing urinometer cylinder and allow it to float freely in it. Make sure it doesn't touch the cylinder's sides.
- Read the mark on the graded scale of the urinometer located at the highest point of the meniscus by levelling the observer's eyes with the surface of the urine. To obtain the corrected specific gravity of the urine sample, specific gravity is usually measured at 15^0C. For every 3^0C difference, 0.001 must be added if the temperature is higher or deducted if it is lower.

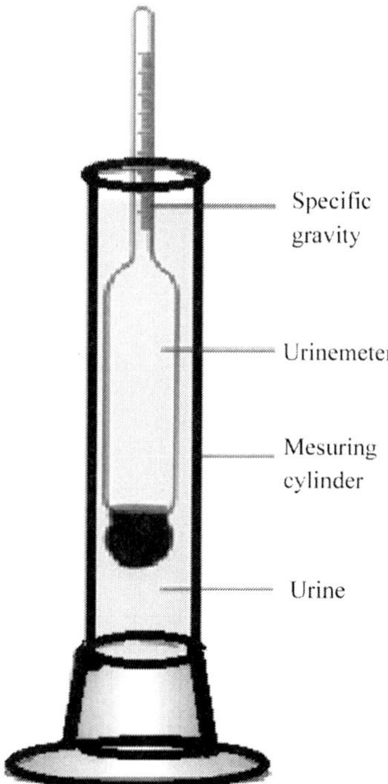

Fig. 5.1: Illustration of the measurement of specific gravity of urine by a Urinometer.

Note: Avoid having air bubbles at the top of the urine samples since they affect how accurately the meniscus is read. It is advisable to occasionally use distilled water to check the urinometer's accuracy. The specific gravity of distilled water at room temperature ought to be 1.000.

B. Refractometer

It is a device that measures the urine's specific gravity based on how many dissolved particles are present. Higher the dissolved particle content, the higher the refractive index, and hence, the higher the specific gravity of the urine.

Procedure

- Pour a drop of freshly voided urine sample on the glass plate of the refractometer.
- Close the plastic cover of the refractometer.
- Take note of the reading on the internal scale.

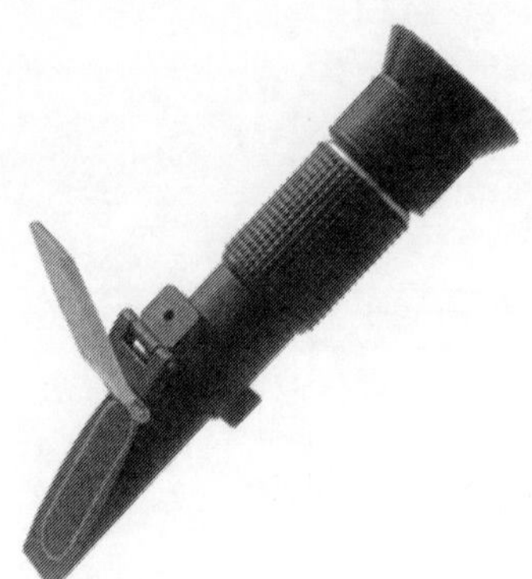

Fig. 5.2: Refractometer.

Note: The specific gravity is influenced by temperature. Therefore, distilled water should be used to calibrate a refractometer before use. Additionally, the device must be dry and clean before usage.

Reference value for specific gravity of urine

In animals, the reference value for urine's specific gravity varies depending on the species (Table 5.4). The specific gravity of urine is also influenced by age, sex, diet, and health.

Table 5.5: Reference intervals for specific gravity in domestic animals:

S. No	Animals	Mean specific gravity (ranges)
1.	Cat	1.030 (1.02-1.040)
2.	Cattle	1.032 (1.030-1.045)
3.	Dog	1.025 (1.016-1.060)
4.	Goat	1.030 (1.015-1.045)
5.	Horse	1.040 (1.025-1.060)
6.	Sheep	1.030 (1.015-1.045)
7.	Swine	1.012 (1.010-1.050)

Increased specific gravity

- Gylocsuria, acute interstitial nephritis, severe vomiting, diarrhoea, fever, reduced feed intake, etc.

Decreased specific gravity

- Advanced stages of uremia, increased fluid intake, the inability of the kidneys to concentrate urine, diabetes insipidus, etc.

5.5. Chemical Analysis of Urine

Urine has typical chemical compositions. However, in pathological conditions or when kidney functions are disrupted owing to damage or infection, urine composition fluctuates in both type and quantity. Urea, creatinine, uric acid, ammonium salts, chlorides, sulfates, and phosphates of sodium, potassium, calcium, and magnesium are generally expelled in urine as ultimate body metabolism waste products. However, glucose, protein, ketone bodies, bilirubin, and bile salts are abnormal urinary components that are discharged in certain renal pathologies. This is why chemical analysis of urine is performed to detect the presence of unusual elements in urine such as glucose, protein, ketone bodies, bile salt, bile pigments, and blood, which aids in the investigation of the individual's health status.

5.5.1.a. Detection of Glucose in Urine

Glucose is the primary sugar in the blood that supplies energy for the metabolic process. When the body wants energy, glucose is oxidized to pyruvate and then to acetyl Co-A to enter the Krebs or Tricarboxylic acid cycle. Normally, urine contains no detectable glucose since the proximal convoluted tubule has reabsorbed nearly all of the glucose molecules contained in the tubular load. As a result, their presence in the urine indicates pathogenic conditions. Glycosuria is the presence of glucose in the urine. The test for detecting glucose in the urine is very beneficial in disease diagnosis. The following are the most often-used laboratory tests for detecting glycosuria in urine:

A. Benedict's test.

B. Fehling's test.

A. Benedict's test

It is a qualitative test. When reducing sugars are heated in the presence of an alkali, they are converted into potent reducing molecules known as 'enediols'. The cupric ion in Benedict's reagent is reduced by enediols to cuprous ions, which precipitate as insoluble red copper oxide. Based on the degree of colour production, the results are graded as nil, 1+, 2+, 3+, and 4+. The amount of reducing sugar in the urine sample determines the degree of colour development. This is the most reliable test because it can detect extremely minute amounts of glucose in a urine sample. This test is not affected by uric acid or creatinine. The overall reaction is summarized below.

$$\text{Cupric ion } (Cu^{2+}) + \text{Reducing sugar} \xrightarrow[\text{Heat}]{\text{Alkali}} \text{Cuprous ions} + \text{Oxidized sugar}$$

Materials required

- Test tubes, pipette, spirit lamp, test tube holder, urine sample, etc.

Reagents

- Spirit and Benedict's reagent.

Benedict's reagent: Dissolve 173 g of sodium citrate and 100g of anhydrous sodium carbonate in 600mL of distilled water in a 1000mL beaker and then warm it gently (solution A). In another beaker, dissolve 17.3g of hydrated $CuSO_4$ in 100mL of distilled water (solution B). Then, add solution B to solution A with constant stirring and make a final volume of 1000mL with distilled water.

Procedure

- Take 5 mL of Benedict's reagent in a test tube.
- Add 8-10 drops of a well-mixed freshly, voided urine sample to the test tube containing Benedict's reagent.
- Then, boil the mixed solution vigorously for 2 minutes and allow it to cool spontaneously.
- Observe the colour change and assign a grade based on the colour of the mixed solution as follows:

S.No	Reaction and colour	Grade	Glucose concentration (mg/dL)
1.	Blue or green without precipitation	Nil	100
2.	Green with yellow precipitation	+	$\geq$ 250
3.	Yellow to olive colour precipitation	++	$\geq$ 800
4.	Brown	+++	$\geq$ 1400
5.	Orange or red	++++	$\geq$ 2000

Fehling's test

Reducing carbohydrates such as glucose, fructose, etc react with alkaline copper sulfate to form the colourful cuprous oxide precipitate. The reactions are summarized below:

$$CuSO_4 + 2KOH \longrightarrow Cu(OH)_2 + K_2SO_4$$

$$\text{Cupric ion } (Cu^{2+}) + \text{Reducing sugar} \xrightarrow[\text{Heat}]{\text{Alkali}} \text{Cuprous ions} + \text{Oxidized sugar}$$

Materials required

- Test tubes, pipette, spirit lamp, test tube holder, urine sample, etc.

Reagents

1. *Fehling's solution A:* Dissolve 69.38 g of copper sulfate in distilled water in a beaker and make the final volume of 1000 mL with distilled water.
2. *Fehling's solution B:* Dissolve 34.6 g of sodium-potassium tartrate (Rochelle's salt) and 20 g of KOH in distilled water, and make the final volume 100 mL with distilled water.

   Mix equal volumes of solution A and solution B just before use.

Procedure

- Take 1 mL of Fehling's solution and 1 mL of urine in a separate test tube.
- Boil the urine and Fehling's solution simultaneously, and then mix them.
- Let the tube cool without further heating.
- Observe the colour change. A brick-red or yellow precipitate indicates that glucose is present in the urine sample.

Note: The Fehling's test is not entirely reliable when used to detect sugar in urine for the following reasons:

- Compounds like conjugated glucuronates, nucleoproteins, etc, when present in sufficient amounts.
- Ammonium salt also interferes with Fehling's test by hindering cuprous oxide precipitation.

Glycosuria

- **Physiological:** After large ingestion of carbohydrate, emotional stress, and pregnancy.

- **Pathological:** Diabetes mellitus, hyperpituitarism, hyperthyroidism, hyperadrenalism, chronic liver disease, enterotoxaemia in sheep and acute and chronic pancreatic necrosis.

Note: The presence of reducing agents like antibiotics, lactose, ascorbic acid, salicylates, morphine, formaldehyde, and uric acid may give a false-positive reaction for glucose.

5.5.1.b. Detection of Proteins in Urine

Protein is a macromolecule made up of one or more polypeptide chains, each with its own sequence of amino acids and molecular weight. Proteins perform a variety of biological functions in the body, including enzyme (e.g., trypsin), transport protein (e.g., haemoglobin, myoglobin), nutrient, storage protein (e.g., ovalbumin (egg), casein (milk), contractile or motile protein (e.g., actin, myosin), structural protein (e.g., keratin, fibroin, collagen), defence protein (e.g., antibodies, fibrinogen), and regulatory protein (e.g., insulin, growth hormone) functions in the body. Normally, these substances do not appear in the urine. Even though only a small amount of protein is filtrated through glomerular capillary tufts, it is reabsorbed by renal tubular cells via pinocytosis. However, if the kidney is damaged, proteins will occur in the urine, depending on the form of the pathological disease. The following are the most often used laboratory tests for determining proteinuria:

A. Robert's test

B. Heat and acetic acid test

C. Sulphosalicylic acid test

D. Heller's ring test

A. Robert's Test

The test is based on protein precipitation from a urine sample using Robert's reagent. The amount of precipitated protein is proportional to the amount of protein contained in the urine sample, and the results are commonly graded as negative, trace, 1+, 2+, 3+, or 4+.

Materials required

- Test tubes, pipette, spirit lamp, test tube holder, urine sample, etc.

Robert's reagent

- Add 200 mL of nitric acid (HNO_3) to 1 liter of saturated magnesium sulfate solution ($MgSO_4$).

Procedure

- Take 2 mL of Robert's reagent in a test tube and then layer 2 mL of urine on top of the reagent by inclining the test tube and letting the urine to run down the side gently with a long dropper or pipette. A white ring at the point of contact indicates the presence of protein in the urine sample.
- Observe the test and note the findings as follows:

Observation	Inference
No ring at the zone of contact	Negative
Distinct narrow ring	+
Wider, definite ring	++
Very wide ring	+++
Thick dense ring occupies most or the entire urine layer	++++

b. Heat and acetic acid test

The test is based on the coagulation of proteins by heat, which causes them to appear cloudy. This approach is the most sensitive, and can detect protein quantities as low as 2 to 3 mg/dL.

Materials required

- Test tubes, pipette, spirit lamp, test tube holder, urine sample, etc.

Reagents

- Glacial acetic acid.

Procedure

- Take about 2 mL of urine in a test tube and boil it for around 2 minutes without shaking.
- The appearance of a white cloud indicates the presence of protein in the urine sample.
- To confirm, add 10 drops of 10 glacial acetic acid drop by drop.
- The persistence of a white cloud implies proteinuria.
- Observe the test and note the findings as follows:

Observation	Inference	Approximate protein concentration (mg/dL)
No turbidity	Negative	-
Perceptible turbidity	Trace	20
Distinct turbidity	+	50
Turbidity with granulation	++	200
Turbidity with granulation and flocculation	+++	500
Clumps of precipitated protein, or solid precipitate	++++	1000

C. Sulphosalicylic acid Test

The test is based on the precipitation of proteins by sulphosalicylic acid, particularly albumin.

Materials required

- Test tubes, pipette, test tube holder and urine sample.

Reagents

- *Sulphosalicylic acid (20% W/v):* Dissolve 200 g of sulphosalcylic acid in distilled water and make the volume 1 liter.

Procedure

- Take 3 mL of urine in a test tube.
- Add 3 mL of 20 % sulphosalicylic acid and mix it thoroughly.
- Observe the appearance of turbidity after 10 minutes, and note the results as follows:

Observation	Inference	Approximate protein concentration (mg/dL)
No turbidity	Negative	-
Perceptible turbidity	Trace	20
Distinct turbidity	+	50
Turbidity with granulation	++	200
Turbidity with granulation and flocculation	+++	500
Clumps of precipitated protein, or solid precipitate	++++	1000

D. Heller's test

The test is based on precipitation of proteins by adding nitric acid to the urine sample. The amount of precipitated protein is proportional to the amount of protein present in the urine. The results are generally graded as negative, trace, 1+, 2+, 3+, or 4+.

Materials required

- Test tubes, pipette, spirit lamp and test tube holder, urine sample, etc.

Reagents

- Nitric acids.

Procedure

- Take 2 mL of nitric acid in a test tube and then layer 2 mL of urine on top of the reagent by inclining the test tube and letting the urine run down the side gently with a long dropper or pipette.
- A white ring at the point of contact indicates the presence of protein in the urine sample.

Note: This test is not suitable for routine proteinuria analysis due to the very corrosive nature of concentrated nitric acid.

Proteinuria

- *Physiological:* Excessive muscular exercise, convulsions, emotional stress, ingestion of an excessive amount of protein and later stage of pregnancy.
- *Pathological:* Glomerulonephritis, tubular dysfunction, hematuria, haemoglobinuria, severe renal diseases, multiple myeloma, leukemia, etc.

5.5.1.c. Detection of Ketone Bodies

Acetoacetic acid and β-hydroxybutyric acid, the two ketone bodies, are difficult to detect in blood or urine. However, if there is insufficient carbohydrate in the diet or a failure in carbohydrate metabolism or absorption, ketone bodies are produced from fat in the liver to act as an alternate fuel for cells. Excess ketone body production and buildup in the body causes ketonemia, which finally manifests in the urine and is known as ketonuria. The following are the most common laboratory tests used to detect ketonuria in urine:

A. Rothera's test

B. Gerhardt's test

A. Rothera's test

Ketone bodies (acetone and acetoacetate) react with an alkaline solution of sodium nitroprusside to form a purple-coloured complex.

Materials required

- Test tubes, pipette, test tube holder, urine sample, etc.

Reagents

- Rothera's reagents and ammonium hydroxide.

Rothera's reagents contains-

Sodium nitroprusside: 0.75 g

Ammonium sulphate: 20g

Procedure

- Take 3 mL of urine in a test tube.
- Add 1 mL of Rothera's reagents and mix it thoroughly.
- Add 1 mL of concentrated ammonium hydroxide solution (28% full strength) on top of the mixture.
- Observe the test. The presence of acetone in the urine sample is indicated by the dark purple colour.

B. Gerhardt's test

Acetoacetate, in particular, reacts with ferric chloride ($FeCI_3$) to produce a Bordeaux-red colour complex.

Materials required

- Test tubes, pipette, test tube holder, urine sample, etc.

Reagents

- *Ferric chloride (10%):* Dissolve 10 g of ferric chloride in distilled water and make the volume 100 mL.

Procedure

- Take 5 mL of urine in a test tube.
- Add 10% mL of ferric chloride solution drop by drop until any precipitate of ferric phosphate dissolves. The presence of acetoacetate is

indicated by the red-brown to Bordeaux red (dark red) colour, although other compounds such as phenol and sodium bicarbonate can provide a similar colour.

- To validate the results, divide the test solution into two equal parts and boil one for 5 minutes. Acetoacetic acid is present if the colour disappears or becomes lighter after boiling.

Ketonuria

- High-fat diet, high fever, starvation, diabetes mellitus in dogs, severe vomiting, diarrhoea, acidosis, impaired liver function, milk fever, and certain endocrine disorders. High fever and starvation may result in ketonuria in puppies and kittens.

5.5.1.d. Detection of Presence of Bilirubin and Biliverdin

Bilirubin is a haemoglobin breakdown product that is transported to the liver by reticuloendothelial cells. In the liver, bilirubin conjugates with glucuronic acid to form bilirubin glucuronide, a water-soluble, stable compound that is eliminated through urine in certain diseases. Urinary bilirubin is usually employed to diagnose liver disease or a hemolytic disorder. The following are the most popular laboratory assays for detecting bilirubin in urine samples:

A. Harrison's (Fouchet's) test

B. Gmelin's test

A. Harrison's (Fouchet's) test

The test is based on the precipitation of bilirubin with barium chloride, which is then oxidized to biliverdin with Fouchet's reagent.

Materials required

- Test tubes, pipette, test tube holder, filter paper, urine sample, etc.

Reagents

- *Barium chloride (10%):* Dissolve 10 g of barium chloride in distilled water and make the volume 100 mL.
- *Fouchet's Reagent*: Dissolve 25 g of trichloroacetic acid in distilled water. Then, add 10 mL of 10% ferric chloride and make the final volume 100 mL with distilled water in a volumetric flask.

Procedure

- Take 10 mL urine sample in a test tube.
- Add 5 mL of a barium chloride solution to the side of the urine test tube and then mix it.
- Allow it to stand for a few minutes.
- Then filter the mixed solution through a small filter paper.
- Take one or two drops of Fouchet's reagent on a dry piece of filter paper and spread it out.
- Observe the colour change. A blue-to-green colour indicates a positive reaction.

Note: The bilirubin test should be performed on fresh urine sample. Because bilirubin is not stable.

B. Gmelin's test

The test is based on the oxidation of bile pigments by acids to coloured derivatives.

Materials and reagent required

- Test tubes, pipette, test tube holder, urine sample, nitric acids, etc.

Procedure

- Take 2 mL of Nitric acid in a test tube.
- Then add 2 mL of urine to it.
- Observe the test. If bilirubin is present, green, blue, or violet rings appear at the liquid-liquid interface.

Increased bile pigments

- Liver disease, hepatocellular disease, hemolytic disease, and bile duct obstruction.

5.5.1.e. Detection of Blood and Haemoglobin in Urine

Hematuria is the presence of intact RBCs in the urine and is consideration to be indicative of bleeding somewhere in the urinary tract. It is generally associated with haemoglobinuria caused by excessive hemolysis of RBCs when the urine has a specific gravity of 1.006 or less or is alkaline. Haemoglobinuria is the presence of free haemoglobin in the urine. Haemoglobinuria can be caused by hemolysis in the bloodstream, in a specific organ, such as the kidney or lower urinary tract, or in the sample itself. The most common laboratory tests are:

A. Benzidine test for analysis of hematuria

B. Guaiac test for analysis of haemoglobinuria

A. Benzidine test

The blood peroxidase enzyme decomposes hydrogen peroxide to release oxygen, which then oxidizes benzidine to give it a blue colour.

Materials required

- Test tubes, pipette, test tube holder, urine sample, etc.

Reagents

- *Saturated benzidine reagent:* Dissolve a sufficient amount of benzidine powder in 5 mL of glacial acetic acid.
- *Hydrogen Peroxide (3%):* Dissolve 3g of hydrogen peroxide powder in distilled water and make the volume 100 mL.

Procedure

- Take 1 mL of saturated benzidine and mix it with 0.3 mL of urine and 0.3 mL of 3% hydrogen peroxide.
- Observe the colour change. The blue colour indicates the presence of blood in the urine sample.

Note: This method is no longer utilized since it is carcinogenic.

B. Guaiac test

The peroxidase enzyme in the haemoglobin molecule liberates oxygen from hydrogen peroxide, and the librated oxygen combines with an organic reagent or chromogen to produce a coloured product. The intensity of the colour is determined by the amount of oxygen and haemoglobin liberated in the urine. When the freed oxygen interacts with an organic reagent, blue or green oxidation products are produced. The overall reactions are summarized below:

O_2 + Organic reagent $\longrightarrow$ Blue or green oxidation products

Materials required

- Test tubes, pipette, test tube holder, urine sample, etc.

Reagents

- Acetic acid, ethanol 95 % and 3 % H_2O_2

Procedure

- Take 4 drops of urine and a few drops of acetic acid in a test tube (T1).
- Add a knife point of Guaiac, 2 mL of 95 % ethanol and 2 mL of 3% H_2O_2 (fresh) in the second test tube (T2). Mix it thoroughly.
- Then, slowly pour the mixed solution (T2) into T1.
- Observe the colour change. Haemoglobin is present in urine if the colour is green or blue.

Haemoglobinuria

- Hemolytic anemia, ingestion of certain drugs, incompatible blood transfusion, sickle cell disease crisis with severe hemolysis, etc.

5.5.2. Microscopic Examination of Urine

The urine often contains a small amount of water as well as solids. The presence of solid substances in urine may suggest renal pathology and an individual's health status. Hence, microscopic evaluation of urine sediment must be included in routine urinalysis. Urine should be analyzed as soon as possible after urination. Delays may cause cell breakdown and the accumulation of amorphous urates or phosphate. The primary goal of microscopic urinalysis is to describe normal and abnormal urine sediments as well as their diagnostic features.

Materials required

- Microscope, glass slide, centrifuge tube, centrifuge machine, coverslip, urine sample, etc.

Procedure

- Take 10 mL of freshly voided urine sample in a centrifuge tube.
- Then centrifuge it at 2500 rpm for 10 minutes and decant the supernatant fluid.
- Tap the centrifuge tube's bottom to dislodge the deposit.

- Place a small drop of sediment from the centrifuge tube on a clean slide.
- Use a coverslip to prevent the formation of air bubbles in the sediment.
- Examine the field under a microscope to identify all solid sedimentary substances (Fig.5.3). Sedimentary materials are classified into two types: organised and unorganised deposits.

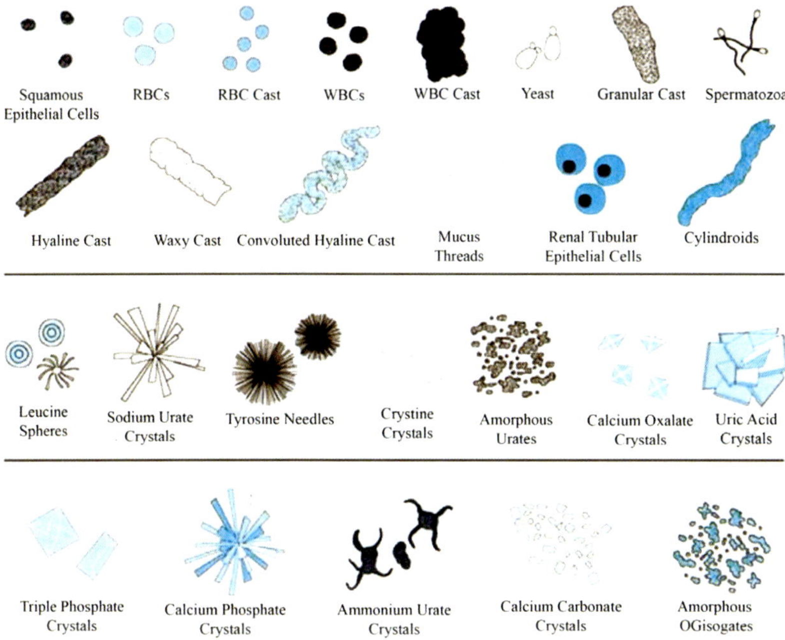

Fig. 5.3: Morphological differences of urine sediment constituents.

Interpretations

Organized sediments: They are formed from living materials	
Organized sediments	***Inference***
Epithelial cells	Increased epithelial cell count in urine samples indicates renal tubular degeneration (acute tubular injury, acute glomerulonephritis, etc.).
Leucocytes	Increased leucocyte counts in urine samples indicate urinary tract infections, all kidney diseases, bladder tumours, etc.
Erythrocytes	An increase in the number of erythrocytes in urine samples indicates the presence of disease conditions in the urinary tract, such as acute and chronic glomerulonephritis, cystitis, kidney injury, etc.
Hyaline casts	The presence of hyaline casts implies that there is minor injury in the urinary system.
Granular casts	The presence of granular casts indicates severe urinary tract injury.

Waxy casts	The presence of granular casts indicates chronic renal disease, tubular inflammation, and degeneration. It is also considered a renal failure cast.
Bacteria	Indicate a urinary tract infection or contamination by genital or intestinal microorganisms.

Yeast cell	**Urinary tract infection.**
Unorganized sediments	The kidney generally secretes crystal-forming substances. Non-living materials such as amorphous urates, uric acid crystals, cystine crystals, calcium phosphate, cholesterol, ammonium biurates, tyrosine, leucine, bilirubin, calcium sulphates (urates), calcium carbonate, calcium oxalate crystals, triple phosphates, amorphous phosphate, calcium carbonate, and calcium phosphate are used to make them. Crystals in urine are determined by the pH, solubility, and concentrations of crystalloids and colloids. Increased calcium oxalate levels suggest a disease state such as diabetes mellitus. Tyrosine and leucine levels that are elevated indicate acute liver damage.

5.6. Determination of Creatinine Concentration in Urine

Creatine phosphate is broken down in the skeletal muscles into creatinine, which is produced almost at a constant rate dependent on muscle mass. This waste product enters the bloodstream and is then removed by the kidneys. Under normal circumstances, this material is easily filtered through the glomeruli of the kidney; the nephron tubules do not reabsorb it. Low levels of creatinine in the urine thus provide a rough indication of renal function. This is why creatinine is such an important biomarker of glomerular filtration rate (GFR) and renal pathology.

The Jaffe reaction is the foundation of the most widely used method for measuring creatinine in urine. In accordance with this, creatinine in protein-free filtrate combines with alkaline picrate to give creatinine picrate a yellow-red colour.

Materials required

- Volumetric flask (100 mL), pipette, reagents, spectrophotometer, urine sample, etc.

Reagents

1. 10 % sodium tungstate.
2. N/10 sulfuric acid (1.15 mL concentrated of sulfuric acid in 500 mL of water).

3. 1 % picric acid solution.
4. 10 % sodium hydroxide solution.
5. 0.1N hydrochloric acid dilutes 4.0 mL of concentrated hydrochloric acid in 500 mL water.
6. Alkaline picrate reagent (mix 5 volumes of picric acid with 1 volume of 10% sodium hydroxide). Always prepare fresh.
7. Standard creatinine solution.

Procedure

- Take two 100 mL volumetric flasks and mark them as "T" (Test) and "B" (Blank).
- Take 0.5 mL of urine and 0.5 mL of distilled water in a "T" flask and only 1 mL of distilled water in a "B" flask.
- Then add 20 mL of 1% Picric acid solution followed by 1.5 mL of 10% Sodium Hydroxide solution to each flask.
- Mix them well and allow them to stand for 15 minutes.
- Read the optical density of the test sample at 520 nm wave lengths after calibrating a spectrophotometer to zero with a blank. Then, calculate the amount of creatinine in the urine from the standard curve.
- The standard curve of creatinine is prepared by taking 0.0, 0.25, 0.50, 0.75, and 1 mL of creatinine solution (1.0 g of dried creatinine dissolved in 1 liter of 0.1N of hydrochloric acid). Treat it with acid and alkali as mentioned above for "T".
- Read the optical density of the standard solutions at 520 nm wavelengths after calibrating a spectrophotometer to zero with a blank. Then, to produce a standard curve, plot a graph of optical density vs creatinine concentration (mg).

Reference value of creatinine level in urine

The reference values of creatinine vary greatly among species in animals.

Table 5.6: Reference intervals for creatinine level in domestic animals:

Species	Cattle	Goat	Sheep	Pig	Dog	Cat
creatinine level (mg/ kg B. wt. day)	15-20	10	10	20-90	30-80	12-20

Low creatinine concentration

- Chronic kidney disease, liver disease, and muscle disease, such as muscular dystrophy. It is also seen in associated with excess water loss, pregnancy, excess water intake, and certain medications.

5.7. Determination of Inorganic Phosphorous in Urine

Phosphorus is an essential mineral, and it is required for intermediate metabolism, skeletal formation, dentition, acid-base balance, and pathological processes such as the genesis of kidney stones. Phosphorus is found as an inorganic phosphate in extracellular fluids. The kidney controls phosphate levels by excreting excess free phosphate from the body through urine. Phosphaturia fluctuations are a natural physiological occurrence. However, chronic phosphate excretion in the urine for more than 24 hours is associated with a pathogenic state. As a result, free phosphate concentration in urine samples is one of the most important indicators of kidney pathology, hormonal abnormalities, and metabolic syndrome.

Methods of estimation of inorganic phosphorous

1. Spectrophotometric or colorimetric method
2. Enzymatic method
3. Chromatographic method
4. Electroanalytical method
5. Other methods that include the classical methods such as gravimetry, titration, etc

The spectrophotometric approach is the most often used method since it is simple to implement and produces accurate results. The test principle is based on the acidic reduction of the phosphomolybdate complex to coloured molybdenum. The colour of the reaction product varies depending on the types of reducing agents used. A spectrophotometer is used to determine the optical density of these reaction color-products. The colour compound's intensity is proportional to the amount of phosphorous in the urine sample.

Materials required

- Measuring cylinder, 100 mL volumetric flask, beaker, pipette, spectrophometer, urine sample collected over 24 hours, etc.

Reagents

- Standard phosphate (0.4 mg/5 mL)
- 2.5 % ammonium molybdate (Molybdate-I)
- 0.25% aminonaphtholsulfonic acid
- 5 N sulfuric acid

Procedure

- Take three volumetric flasks (100 mL capacity) and mark them as "T" (unknown/test) (T), "S" (standard), and "B" (blank).
- Take reagents, test sample and standard into all marked flasks as follows:

Reagents / Sample / Urine/ Distilled water	T-flask	S-flask	B-flask
Urine	Enough urine which contain between 0.2 and 0.8 mg of inorganic phosphate	Nil	Nil
Distilled water (mL)	Upto 70	65	70
Ammonium molybdate (2.5%) or Molybdate-I (mL)	10	10	10
Aminonaphtholsulfonic acid (0.5%) in mL	4	4	4
Standard phosphate solution (mL)	-	5	-
Distilled water	Up to 100	Up to 100	Up to 100

- Gently shake the tubes to mix them properly. Incubate the solution for 5 minutes at room temperature.
- Read the optical density of the samples and standard, against the blank in a spectrophotometer at 660 to 720 nm, after setting to zero density with the blank.
- Calculate the inorganic phosphate in the urine sample using the following formula:
- Inorganic phosphate (mg) in the volume of urine =

$$\frac{O.D.\ unknown\ /\ Test\ sample\ (T)}{O.D.\ standard} X\ 0.4$$

Hypophosphaturia

- Rachitism
- Osteomalacia
- Hypovitaminosis D
- Idiopathic steatorrhea
- Renal hyperparathyroidism
- Hypohypoparathyroidism
- Pseudohypoparathyroidism
- Chronic renal failure

Hyperphosphaturia

- Myeloma
- Vitamin D intoxication
- Fanconi's syndrome
- Nephritis
- Renal rickets

5.8. Determination of Total Titrable Acidity

The kidneys regulate the body's acid-base balance by excreting acids into the urine. The renal net total acid excretion and retention capacity are affected by the dietary acid load. This is why measuring renal total acid excretion is used to assess kidney pathology.

This test in urine is based on the amount of alkali required to change the pH from the original value to the phenolphthalein endpoint pH as an indication.

Materials required

- Burette, pipette, conical flask, urine sample, etc.

Reagent

- 0.1 N NaOH solution, 1% phenolphthalein solution and potassium oxalate.

Procedure

- Take 25 mL of urine in a conical flask.
- Add 5 g of potassium oxalate (freshly prepared powder) and 0.5 mL of Phenolphthalein solution to the flask containing the urine sample.
- Mix the solution by shaking vigorously.
- Then, titrate immediately with 0.1 N NaOH solutions until a pink colour develops. The pink colour lasts only approximately a minute.
- Repeat the experiment three times and compute the mean of the three time values.
- Calculate the total titrable acidity of the urine sample using the formula below.

$$\frac{25}{A} x \frac{B}{X}$$

Therefore,

$$X = \frac{A \text{ x } B}{25}$$

Where,

A = mL of 0.1N NaOH solution used.

B = volume of urine excreted in 24 hours.

X = Total acidity in urine sample.

Tirable acidity in the samples is expressed in mEq/24 hours.

5.9. Terminology

- Anuria: A complete cessation of micturition.
- Diuresis: An increased or excessive production of urine.
- Oliguria: A reduction in urine output.
- Polyuria: Excessive urine production or urine output.
- Dysuria: Difficult or painful micturition.
- Stranguria: Slow, dropwise, and painful micturition.
- Glycaemia: A high level of sugar in the blood.
- Glycosuria: The presence of sugar in the urine.
- Haemoglobinuria: The presence of haemoglobin in the urine.

- Haematuria: The presence of intact red blood cells in the urine.
- Ketonaemia: The presence of ketone bodies in the blood.
- Ketonuria: The presence of ketone bodies in the urine.
- Renal calculus: A stone in the kidney.

6

Endocrine System Hormone Bioassays

6.0. Introduction

Endocrinology is the study of the endocrine system, which includes the glands and their secretions known as hormones. Hormones are essential for animal behaviour, growth and development, metabolism, lactation, reproduction, excretion, and reabsorption of inorganic ions. Therefore, if a certain hormone concentration in blood or another body fluid is detected, it provides the pathophysiology of the representative endocrine gland.

Endocrine glands, the cells or tissues they govern, and the secretory substances (hormones) they produce are investigated using a number of methodologies. They are as follows:

1. Surgical methods (e.g., hypophysectomy, gonadectomy, etc).
2. Chemical ablation or impairment (e.g., alloxan or streptozotocin agents that selectively destroy the insulin-secreting beta-cell, etc).
3. Hormone replacement therapy (e.g., estrogen during menopause to reduce the risk of bone fracture related to osteoporosis, etc).
4. Immunological neutralization of hormone activity (e.g., contraception both male and female, injection of antibodies against NGF resulting in failure of sympathetic nervous system development, etc).
5. Tissue extraction and purification (e.g., progestin is a synthetic hormone that mimics progesterone, etc.).
6. Histological-cytological studies (e.g., employment of a battery of histological stains to characterize each pituitary cell, etc).
7. Bioassays (e.g., oxytocin-induced contraction of rat uterine myometrial tissue strips, etc).

6.1. Bioassay for Trophic Hormones

The physiological activity of a hormone was initially determined using the bioassay approach, in which the biological activity of a hormone is investigated in living cells, tissues, or organs that are naturally sensitive to the hormone. The bioassay can be performed *in vitro* or *in vivo*. Almost all hormones have bioassays based on their functional and physiological action in the specified living cells, tissues, or organs. For example, the uterotrophic bioassay for estrogen in immature rats or mice is a reliable, easy, and extremely sensitive test, thyroxine-induced metamorphosis in tadpoles, etc.

6.2. Bioassay for Estrogen in Immature Mice or Rats

The test is based on a dose-dependent increase in uterine weight to body weight ratio in response to subcutaneous injections of 17β-estradiol (0.1–500μg/kg/day) for three consecutive days in immature female mice or rats. Estrogen induces increases in cell proliferation and macromolecule synthesis, which cause uterine weight gain.

Materials required

- Weighing balance, needle and syringe, immature female rats, 17β-estradiol, etc.

Procedure

- Select twenty immature female rats. Then divide them into five groups (n=4 in each group) as control (C) and treatment groups (T1, T2, T3, and T4).
- Take note of the rat's body weight (pre-17β-estradiol injection weight).
- Inject 17β-estradiol dissolved in corn oil into all rats of the T1, T2, T3, and T4 groups for three consecutive days subcutaneously at a dose rate of 1, 10, 100, or 500μg/kg/day, and only 0.1 mL of corn oil to all female rats of the control group.
- Measure the weight of each rat the day after the final injection. The rats are then sacrificed by cervical dislocation, and the uterus is meticulously dissected to recover an intact wet uterus.
- Measure the weight of an intact wet uterus for each rat.
- Calculate the % uterine weight of each rat as follows:

$$\% \text{ Binding} = \frac{\text{CPM(Sample or standard)-NSB}}{\text{CPM}\left(\text{Maximum binding}\right)\text{-NSB}} \text{ X } 100$$

Table 6.1: Bioassay of estrogen in rats

Group	Average body weight after treatment	Average weight of the intact wet uterus	Increase in weight	% increase in weight
Control Treatment groups T1 T2 T3 T4				

6.3. Immunoassay

Hormones are found in trace amounts in the circulating blood. It was difficult to measure hormone levels at the beginning of endocrinology. Rosalyn Yalow and Solomon Berson invented the groundbreaking method known as radioimmunoassay in the middle of the 20th century (1950s), which makes it feasible to quantify hormones and their byproducts. Lately several immunoassay approaches have been developed in an effort to improve the sensitivity, specificity, accuracy, and reliability of measuring hormone concentrations in body fluids. The basis of an immunoassay is the utilization of antibody and antigen complexes to provide a quantifiable result. They are as follows:

1. Radioimmunoassay (RIA)
2. Enzyme-Linked Immunosorbent Assays (ELISA)
3. Fluoroimmunoassay (FIA)
4. Chemiluminescence immunoassay (CLIA)

6.4. Estimation of Progesterone in Plasma

Hormone concentrations in blood or other body fluids are frequently quantified by RIA. This technique has enabled the quantification of hormones in extremely low quantities with high specificity.

Principle of RIA

The hormone or unlabeled hormone or antigen [H] (to be quantified) competes for limited binding sites on a specific antibody [Ab] produced against the hormone or antigen to be quantified. The concentration of radiolabeled hormone [H*] is indirectly determined by measuring the concentration of unlabeled hormone [H]. Because the levels of radiolabeled hormone [H*] and antibodies [Ab] are fixed. The overall reactions are as follows:

[H]+ [Ab] ⟶ [H] [Ab]

[H*] + [H] [Ab] ⟶ [H] [Ab] + [H*][Ab]

Estimation of Progesterone by RIA

1. Materials required

- Assay tubes, weighing balance, beakers, pipettes, scintillation vials, and β-counter or γ-gamma counter, vortex, and water bath.

Reagents

- Assay buffer (dissolves 69 g of KH_2PO_4, 8.3 g of Na_2HPO_4, 8.5 g of NaCI, 0.1 g of thimerosal, and 1.0 g of gelatin in distilled water and makes a volume of 1000 mL), radiochemical, or tracer (progesterone I^{125}). Antiserum for progesterone, progesterone standard, diethyl ether, ice salt, and plasma samples.

Procedure

1. Extraction of plasma samples with the ethanol:
   - Take 200 μL of plasma samples and 2 mL of chilled diethyl-ether in duplicate test tubes and vortex them for 1 minute.
   - Keep the test tubes in an ice-salt mixture to freeze the lower aqueous layer.
   - Decant the top ether layer from each test tube to another tube. Extraction should be repeated with cold diethyl ether.
   - Then, put the test tubes in a water bath to evaporate the 4.0 mL of ether to dryness.
   - Add 1 mL of ether to all tubes and vortex them for 30 seconds to wash the hormone from the walls of the test tubes. Again, evaporate to dryness by placing the tubes in a water bath.
   - After drying, add 200 μL of assay buffer to all test tubes and vortex it for 30 seconds.
   - Then incubate all tubes at 50°C for one hour in a water bath, followed by a vortex for 30 seconds (for ethanol-extracted plasma samples).
2. Prepare the progesterone standard (containing progesterone in concentrations ranging from 0.1 to 60 ng/100L) as follows:

- Dissolve 16 mg of progesterone in ethanol and make the volume 100 mL. This stock solution will have a progesterone concentration of 16 μg/100μL (stock A).
- Take 100 μL of stock A and evaporate it to dryness by placing it in a water bath. Then, add 100 mL of ethanol to the dry test tube (stock B). The stock B solution has a progesterone concentration of 160 ng/mL. Stock B is used for assays as mentioned in protocols.

3. Perform the assay in accordance with the procedure mentioned below:

Scintillation vials	**Name**	**Tracer (μL)**	**Antibody (μL)**	**Standard or sample (μL)**	**Assay Buffer(μL)**
1-2	TC	100	-	-	-
3-4	NSB	100	-	-	400
5-6	MB Zero std	100	100	-	300
7-8	0.1 ng	100	100	100	200
9-10	0.3 ng	100	100	100	200
11-12	0.6 ng	100	100	100	200
13-14	1.0 ng	100	100	100	200
15-16	5.0 ng	100	100	100	200
17-18	20.0 ng	100	100	100	200
19-20	40.0 ng	100	100	100	200
21-22	60.0 ng	100	100	100	200
23-24	Sample	100	100	200 μL assay buffer	100
25	QC	100	100	200 μL assay buffer	100

4 Vortex the reaction mixture and keep the scintillation vials at room temperature overnight.

5. Add 1.0 mL polyethylene glycol to each scintillation vial except TC. It must separate the free and bound fractions of the reaction mixtures.

6. Incubate all scintillation vials at 4°C for 1 hour after vortexing.

7. Centrifuge all tubes at 200 g for 45 minutes. Then decant all scintillation vials and leave them inverted over absorbent paper for 30 minutes to ensure that the last few drops of the reaction mixture are removed.

8. Count the CPM in tubes using a β-counter.

9. Calculate the % binding for the standard and samples as follows:

$$\%\ \text{Binding} = \frac{\text{CPM(Sample or standard)-NSB}}{\text{CPM}\left(\text{Maximum binding}\right)\text{-NSB}} \text{ X } 100$$

10. Plot a standard curve with the standard on X-axis and % binding on Y-axis.
11. Compute the concentration of test samples by interpolating on the standard curve and expressing the results in ng/mL.

6.5. Estimation of Estrogen in Plasma

A modified version of RIA is the enzyme-linked immunosorbent assay (ELISA). Instead of radioisotopes, a stable enzyme is used to label or conjugate hormones.

Principle of ELISA

Estrogens in plasma compete with a fixed amount of estrogens enzyme conjugate for the limited (fixed) estrogen antibody binding sites on the surface of the ELISA plate walls. The amount of bound estrogens enzyme conjugate is determined after adding an enzyme substrate solution based on the optical density (O.D.) of the colour development. The concentration of estrogens in plasma is inversely related to the amount of estrogen enzyme conjugates binding to estrogen antibodies.

Materials required

- ELISA plates (96 well flat bottomed wells), ELISA reader, test tubes, vortex, shaker, micro pipette, 12 channels micropipette, etc.

Reagents

- Benzene
- Antiserum for estrogens
- Goat anti rabbit IgG
- EIA assay buffer –It contains 50 mM NaH_2PO_4/ Na_2HPO_4, 0.15 M NaCl, and 0.1 % bovine serum albumin with a pH of 7.2.
- Washing solution- 0.05% Tween 20.
- Stop solution -4N H_2SO_4.
- Solution A- Dissolve 2 mg of estradiol-17b-glucuronide in 50 µL of methanol and 20 µL of 1 N HCl at 50°C for 2 hours. Then add 500 µL of N, N-dimethyl-formamide, and 6.25 µL of 4-methylmorpholine. Cool the solution to -15^{0}C.

- Solution B- Add 375 μL of dimethyl formamide slowly to 500 μL of Horseradish peroxidase (4.75 mg Horseradish peroxidase /mL of water) and then cool the solution to 0^0C.
- Coating buffer- It contains 15 mM Na_2CO_3 and 35 mM $NaHCO_3$with a pH of 9.6.
- Substrate buffer- It contains 0.05 M citric acid, 0.11M Na_2HPO_4, 0.05% ureumperoxide with a pH of 4.
- Substrate solution- It contains 17 mL of substrate buffer and 340μl of 3,3, 5,5 tetramethyl benzidine.

Procedure

1. Extraction of plasma samples with benzene according to the procedure outlined below:
   - Take 0.5 mL of plasma samples and 3 mL of benzene in a test tube and vortex them for 2 minutes.
   - Pipette out 2.5 mL of the upper organic layer and then evaporate until dry in a hot air oven at 50°C.
   - Then, dissolve the dry test tube residue in 150 mL of EIA assay buffer and vortex it for 30 seconds for complete solubilization (benzene-extracted plasma samples).
2. Prepare the enzyme label (Horseradish peroxidase) for coupling with estradiol-17 β -glucuronide as follows:
   - Add 0.63 mg of goat lgG dissolved in 100 mL of coating buffer per well of the microtiter plate or ELISA plate.
   - Incubate the plate overnight at 4°C (first coating).
   - Add 300 mL of 'EIA assay buffer' containing 1% bovine serum albumin to all the wells of the plate.
   - Again incubate the plate at room temperature for 40 to 50 minutes with constant shaking (second coating).
   - Wash the plates twice with 350 mL of the washing solution.
3. Perform the assay as per the procedure mentioned below:
   - Dispense 50 μL of benzene-extracted plasma samples and estradiol-17-β standards ranging from 0.2 to 100 pg/50 mL prepared in EIA assay buffer into respective wells of the plate, along with 100 mL of

enzyme conjugates diluted in 'EIA assay buffer' at the rates of 1:30,000 and 1:5,000 for total estrogen and estradiol-17β, respectively.

- Then, add 100 mL of antiserum for estrogens diluted in 'EIA assay buffer to each well of the plate except the blank.
- Incubate the plates overnight at 4ºC after 30 minutes of constant agitation in the dark room.
- Wash the plate four times with the washing solution before incubating it for 40 minutes in the dark at room temperature with 150 mL of the substrate solution.
- Add 50 μL of stop solution and read the micro plate with a micro plate reader or ELISA reader at 450 nm.
- Plot a standard curve with the standard on X-axis and % binding on Y-axis.
- Compute the concentration of test samples by interpolating on the standard curve.

6.6. Terminology

- **Accuracy**: It is the extent to which the measurement of a hormone in the sample agrees with the amount added.
- **Specificity**: It is the extent of freedom from interference by substances other than the one intended to be measured.
- **Sensitivity:** It is defined as the lowest concentration of antigen that can be distinguished.
- **Precision:** It is the degree to which the number of measurements of an antigen agrees with the mean concentration.
- **Recovery:** It is the extent to which the amount of hormone measured in a sample corresponds to the exact amount added.
- **NSB (Non-specific binding):** These tubes contain antibodies but no antigen. The non-specific binding of antibodies to other components in the solution causes the reading of these tubes.
- **Titre test:** The titre test determines what concentration or dilution of antigen or antibody is optimal for the interaction to occur and the result produced when counts/O.D. is maximal.

- **Standards:** Standards are tubes containing a known amount of unlabeled antigen. The first set of tubes has the least amount of unlabeled antigen. The following set of tubes has a higher concentration of unlabeled antigen as a result of successive dilutions of the highest concentration of the assay's standard. The lowest and maximum concentrations established for the assay's limits are chosen so that the experimental or predicted values fall between these limits.

7

Physiology of Reproduction

Bhabesh Mili and Tukheswar Chutia

7.0. Introduction

Reproduction is the biological process that results in the formation of new progeny or individual organisms. Male and female gametes unite to form a zygote, which develops or produces offspring.

7.1. Physiology of Female Reproduction

The main female reproductive functions are the production of gametes, or ova (singular=ovum), providing an environment for the fertilization of those ova, nourishment of the embryo & fetus, and finally, providing a mechanism for birth or parturition. Ovum contributes half of the offspring's genetic makeup. The ovum size is about 110-120 μM in diameter. An oocyte is surrounded by a single layer of flattened cells (primordial follicles). The oocyte is an immature female gamete that grows into an ovum during the estrus cycle. Intra-ovarian and extra-ovarian hormones in the ovaries promote the development of oogonium (germ cells) and primordial follicles into the ovum and graafian follicles, or preovulatory follicles.

The cortex of the ovary contains ovarian follicles. Ovarian follicles are categorized into three types based on their developmental stages: (a) Primordial (also known as primary follicles), (b) Growing follicles, and (c) Graafian follicles. The formation of Graafian follicles from a pool of primordial follicles is known as folliculogenesis. It is a very dynamic and rapid process that occurs during the follicular phase of the estrus cycle. FSH is released prior to the recruitment of a cohort of follicles from the pool of primordial follicles. Only GnRH-dependent primordial follicles recruit throughout the follicular phase. Follicles develop in wave patterns and vary widely among animals (Table7.1). LH enhances follicle growth as well as ovum maturation. The growing follicle is composed of developing granulose cells (GC) and a zona pellucid layer, but no theca cell layer or antrum. Garrafian follicles have an antrum, which is a fluid-filled hollow surrounded by two layers of theca (theca interna and theca externa). LH stimulates the granulosa cells to produce estrogen in the follicle. Estrogen triggers a steady increase in LH levels. The ovulatory phase begins with an increase in LH release, which eventually leads to ovulation.

Table 7.1: Follicular diameters and follicular waves in domestic animals:

Animals	LH receptors in GC (Follicular diameter)	Folliculardiameter	Follicular waves
Ewe	4 mm	6-7mm	2-5
Sow	5-6 mm	8-10 mm	No evidence
Cow	8 mm	15-20 mm	2-3
Mare	25 mm	35-50 mm	1-2

The ovarian follicle develops synchronously with the oocyte's mitosis and meiosis divisions. The process by which female primordial germ cells (oogonium) transform into a mature ovum or egg is known as oogenesis (Fig. 7.1). The oocyte of a primordial follicle is a primary oocyte that remains in an arrested stage of meiosis during follicular development. Except for mares, most domestic animals undergo the first meiotic division to form secondary oocytes and the first polar body immediately before ovulation. The first meiotic division occurs in the mare shortly after ovulation. The first polar body is extruded from the ovary. When ovulation occurs, secondary oocytes resume meiosis division and produce haploid oocytes. In most domestic species (cow, ewe, and sow), ovulation occurs as secondary oocytes, except bitch.

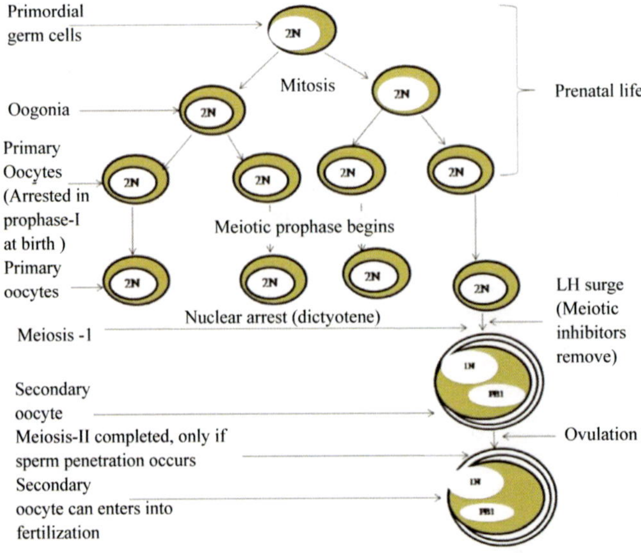

Fig. 7.1: Diagrammatic illustration of the major steps of oogenesis

7.2. Characterization of Mammalian Oocytes

Materials required

- Slaughter house derived ovaries, needle, syringe and stereo-zoom microscope.

Reagents

- Oocyte collection media comprise of 5% bovine serum albumin and 5% fetal calf serum (FCS). Oocytes are also harvested using 3% inactivated FCS in modified phosphate-buffered saline and TCM-199 media with 3% FCS.

Procedure

1. Oocyte collection

Oocytes can be collected from ovaries by four methods viz.,

1. Aspiration method
2. Follicle dissection method
3. Slicing method
4. Ultrasound-guided ovum pickup from live animals

Among all methods, the aspiration method is the relatively best for retrieving quality oocytes. It is also the most preferred method for oocyte collection from slaughter house ovaries.

- Aspirate the mature follicle from the ovary using a sterile plastic syringe (5 or 10-mL volume) and an 18 gauge hypodermic needle. In general, the needle and syringe should be primed with 0.25 or 0.50 mL of normal saline solution or oocyte collection media.
- Then, gently transfer the contents of the syringe into a sterile 50-mL tube after aspiration to avoid disrupting the cumulus-oocyte complex (COCs).
- Allow them to stand for about 15 minutes to settle the oocytes at the bottom of the tube.
- Discard the supernatant without disturbing the sediments or precipitation. The sediments should then be poured into a Petri dish for subsequent oocyte searches under a stereo-zoom microscope.

2. Grading of oocytes

- Examine the characteristics of oocytes under a stereo-zoom microscope and grade them as follows:

Grade	Oocyte characteristics
Grade A	• Compact COCs with an unexpanded cumulus. • ≥ 5 layers of cumulus cells. • Homogenous granular cytoplasm.
Grade B	• ≤ 5 layers of compact cumulus mass. • Homogenous granular cytoplasm.
Grade C	• COCs with 3 layers of cumulus cells. • Homogenous granular cytoplasm.
Grade D	• Without cumulus cell layers. • Irregular cytoplasm.

Note: It is suggested that only grade A and B oocytes be used for *in vitro* fertilization (IVF) and *in vitro* embryo culture (IVC).

7.3. Detection of Estrus in domestic animals

Estrus, also referred to as "heat," is a stage of the reproductive or estrus cycle in which female animals become sexually receptive, signalling that they are ready for mating. This phenomenon develops as a result of the unique action of ovarian steroid hormones. During the last three or four days of an estrus cycle, Graafian follicles synthesize and secrete increasing amounts of estrogen. High eestrogen levels, followed by a surge of LH, trigger ovulation and the manifestation of estrus-related behavioural signs (Fig.7.2). These behavioural signs make sense to identify estrus in female farm animals. It is often performed for planned insemination programmes and the successful use of assisted reproductive technologies. The duration of estrus and the time of ovulation in relation to the commencement of estrus differ between species (Table 7.2).

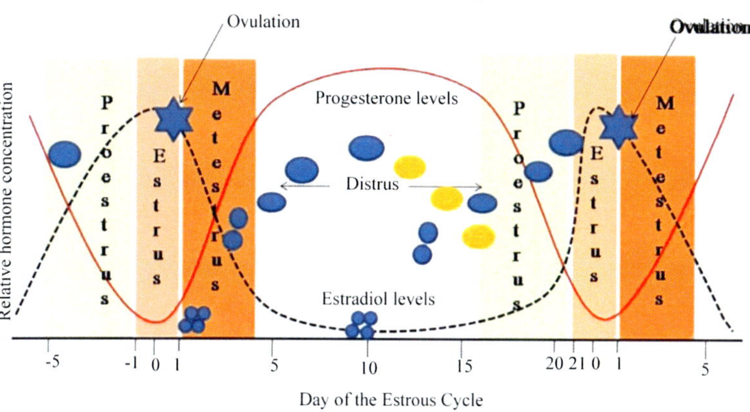

Fig. 7.2: Circulatory hormone patterns associated with follicular growth and ovulation during one estrous cycle in dairy cows.

Table 7.2: Average lengths of various parts of the reproductive cycles in domestic animals:

Animals	Types of estruscycles	Length of estrus cycle (days)	Duration of estrus	Time of ovulation
Cow	Polyestrous	19-23 Average:21	6-30 hours Average: 18 hours	12 hours after end of estrus.
Doe	Seasonal polyestrous in Fall	12-24 Average:20	1-4 days Average: 39 hours	30-36 hours after startof estrus.
Ewe	Seasonal polyestrous in Fall	14-20 Average:17	20-42 hours Average: 30 hours	At or near the end of estrus.
Mare	Seasonal polyestrous in Spring	10-37 Average:21	2 – 6 days Average: 4 days	24-48 hours before the start of estrus to 24 hours after the endof estrus.
Sow	Polyestrous	18-24 Average:21	1– 2 days Average:36 hours	8-12 hours before the end of estrus or 37-40hours after start of estrus.
Bitch	Monestrous	7-8 months interval depending on breed	4 to 24 days Average: 7-9 days	Day 3-6 of estrus.
Queen	Seasonal polyestrous and a long a day breeder	16	5-6 days	Induced 24-32 hours after coitus.

Methods of Estrus Detection

A. Estrus detection based on physical and behavioral signs.

B. Cervical mucus test.

C. Other methods using estrus detection aids that include the use of marker animals, teaser animals, electronic heat-detection aids, electronic pedometers or motion sensors, and the use of milk or blood progesterone assay kits, etc.

7.4.a. Estrus Detection Based on Physical and Behavioral Signs

This method is the simplest way to detect estrus in farm animals. Many species exhibit physical and behavioural signs of estrus, which vary according to the species (Table 7.3). As a result, competent personnel capable of recognizing physical and behavioural signs of estrus are needed.

Procedure

- Ensure that all the animals in the herd are clearly visible from a distance.
- Observe the manifestation of physical and behavioural signs of estrus for two hours after milking in the morning and two hours in the afternoon.
- Take notes on the physical and behavioural signs.

Table 7.3: Physical and behavioral signs of estrus in various animals:

S.No.	Animals	Physical and behavioral signs of estrus
	Cow	• Nervousness and restlessness. • Drop in milk yield and appetite. • Frequent urination. • Red and swollen valve. • Try to mount other animals not in heat. • Clear mucus discharge from the vulva. • Isolation from the herd. • Bawling when isolated. • Allow other animals to mount her. • Scruff marks or dirt from the hooves and saliva on her back. • Ruffled hair near the tail head. • Turn the tail to one side.
	Doe	The signs of estrus are very similar to those observed in cattle. • Seeking out the male. • Constant vocalizations. • Loss of appetite. • Restlessness. • Wagging of tail. • Rubbing up against herd-mates. • Redness and swelling around the vulva. • Thin mucus discharge from the vulva.

S.No.	Animals	Physical and behavioral signs of estrus
	Ewe	• Search-out the ram. • Rapid tail movement or raised tail in the presence of the ram. • Nervousness. • Vocalization for the ram. • Drop in milk production and appetite. • Standing to be mounted by ram or other ewes. • Red and swollen valve.
	Mare	• Seeking out the company of other mares, geldings, and handlers. • Winking of the vulva. • Frequent urination. • Squatting or lowering of the pelvis. • Hind legs spread. • Lifting of the tail.
	Animals	Physical and behavioral signs of estrus
	Sow	• Frequent urination. • Allow another sow or boar to mount her. • Mounting and nudging other females. • Increase vocalizations. • Erect ears in the presence of boar. • Desire to seek out the boar. • Loss of appetite. • Red and swollen vulva. • Increase in vaginal secretions. • Arching of back or lordosis
	Queen	• Increase vocalization (crouching and heat cry sound). • Exhibit lordosis in response to stroking the flanks. • Exhibit treading (short, quick hind limbs extension).
	Bitch	• Hyper excitement. • Frequent urination. • Seeking out for the male. • Reduce appetite. • Sanguineous discharge from a swollen vulva. • Exhibit lordosis in response to male.

7.4.b. Estrus Detection Based on Cervical Mucus Test

Mucus is formed in the cervix and accumulates with other fluids in the vagina before, during, and shortly after estrus in response to high circulatory estrogen levels during the estrus phase. The qualities and quantity of cervix secretion, or mucus, fluctuate depending on the hormone predominance, which corresponds to the period of the estrus cycle. The cervical mucus test is divided into two parts: (1) macroscopic evaluations of the appearance and consistency of mucus and (2) microscopical studies of the arborization pattern of mucus.

7.4 b.1 Macroscopic Examination

- Aspirate cervical mucus from the mid-cervix on the day of estrus, prior to artificial insemination, using a blue sterile sheath and universal AI gun through the recto-vaginal method.
- Then, examine visually for appearance (clear, cloudy, and dirty) and consistency (thick, medium, and watery).
- Take note of the observation.

Indication / interpretation

- Copious mucus and long viscous, clear elastic strands of mucus hanging from the vulva are signs of estrus.
- In heifers, cloudy mucus secretions indicate either late estrus or infection.
- Thick mucus is a sign of good sexual health.
- Dirty mucus discharge indicates uterine infection.

7.4 b.2 Microscopic Examination

The test is based on examining the ferning pattern of cervical mucus with a low-power microscope objective. High chloride level is associated with cervical mucus fern patterns.

Materials required

- Glass slide, microscope, and cervical mucus.

Procedure

- Collect the cervical mucus on the day of estrus prior to the artificial insemination.
- Place a few drops of a well-mixed cervical mucus sample on a grease-free glass slide, spread it evenly, and let it to air dry.
- Examine the air-dried slide under a microscope using a low-power objective (10x) for the crystallization pattern of the mucus, which is known as the fern pattern.
- Observe the degree of ferning, and evaluate them as follows:

    1. Linear ferning only (little estrogen effect).

2. Arborization of leaves at 90 degrees to each other give the appearance of a palm leaf.

3+ Moderate degree of arborization when palm leaf appearance involves angulation at three right angles.

4+ Maximal arborizations with palm leaves arranged at four right angles to one another.

Indication

- The cervical mucus test aids in determining the best timing to inseminate farm animals. During estrus, it is recommended to inseminate farm animals with high-quality sperm, specifically cervical mucus fern patterns with 1 to 2 degrees of arborization.

7.5. Study of Estrus Cycle in Rats by Vaginal Cytology

The basis of this test is the identifying the type of cells present in the vaginal smears. During the estrus cycle, the types of vaginal epithelium change according to estrogen and progesterone levels. Elevated estrogen hormone causes vaginal epithelium to become squamous or cornified, which can be viewed under a microscope after staining a vaginal smear with either Leishman's or Giemsa stain.

Materials required

- Non pregnant adult female rats, thin wooden sticks, cotton, glass slides, staining rack, and microscope, etc.

Reagents

- Normal saline and Leishman's stain or Giemsa stain.

Procedure

- Prepare small, thin cotton buds by wrapping one end of a thin stick.
- Then, dip the cotton bud end of the thin stick in a normal saline solution.
- After securing the rat in your left hand, gently insert a wet tiny cotton bud into the rat's vagina.
- Rotate it once and then remove it.
- Rub or roll the bud on a clean glass slide to prepare a smear.
- Dry the smear in the air.

- Place the air-dried smear on the staining rack and stain it (with either Leishman's or Giemsa stain depending on availability) as described above in Differential Leucocyte Count in Chapter 1.
- Examine the stained smear using low-power objective of a microscope.
- Identify the cells in the stained smear. Determine the stage of the estrus cycle based on the type of cells, as stated in Table 7.4.

Table 7.4: Prediction of the stage of estrus cycle based on vaginal smear cytology in rats:

Vaginal smear cytology	Prediction of the stage estrus cycle
Nucleated epithelial cells dominate the smear.	Proestrus
Cornified (dead) epithelial cells dominate the smear.	Estrus
The smear contains not only cornified epithelial cells, but also leukocytes and some nucleated epithelial cells.	Metestrus
Leukocytes predominate in the smear.	Diestrus

7.6. Physiology of Male Reproduction

The primary functions of male reproduction are the formation of male gametes (sperm or spermatozoa) and the deposition of the gamete into the female reproductive tract during mating. Sperm is a special cell that can move to the female reproductive tract and fertilize an ovum. The testis has two key functions in male reproduction: spermatogenesis and endocrine function. The seminiferous tubules of the testis are the site of spermatozoa's genesis (spermatogenesis).

Spermatogenesis is the process through which germ cells multiply and differentiate into spermatozoa. There are three stages to this process: spermatocytogenesis, meiosis, and spermiogenesis (Fig.7.3). In the initial stage of spermatogenesis, germ cells undergo a series of mitotic divisions that result in spermatogonia and primary spermatocytes. Primary spermatocytes divide by meiosis, which involves genetic material duplication and exchange as well as two cell divisions that reduce the chromosome number and result in four haploid round spermatids. The first meiotic division includes reducing the number of chromosomes and dividing homologous chromosomes, whereas the second meiotic division involves the separation of daughter chromatids. Spermiogenesis is the process by which round spermatids develop into fully developed spermatozoa that are released into the lumen of seminiferous tubules.

Exocrine function, specifically intra- and extra-testicular hormones, aids in the transition of germ cells to spermatozoa (haploid chromosomes), which are released into the lumen of the seminiferous tubules and then released in the epididymis. The endocrine functions are accomplished by Leydig cells and Sertoli cells.

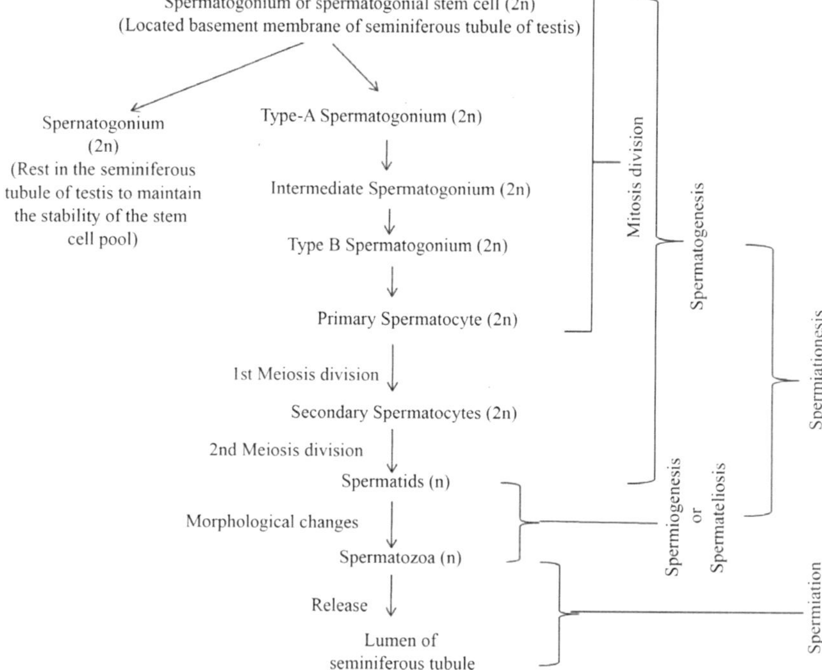

Fig. 7.3: Diagrammatic illustration of the stages of spermatogenesis in mammals

Leydig and Sertoli cells are essential for spermatogenesis. Leydig cells reside in the interstitial spaces of the seminiferous tubules. This cell produces testosterone when stimulated by LH. Testosterone, a male androgen, is required for spermatogenesis, particularly meiosis division, as well as male sexual characteristics such as the development and maintenance of libido, the secretory activity of male accessory glands, the development of resident muscle mass, and other secondary sexual behaviours.

FSH influences Sertoli cell activity, which is essential for the completion of meiosis in germ cells. Under the influence of FSH, the Sertoli cell secretes enzymes that convert testosterone to dihydrotestosterone (DHT), an androgen that stimulates the development of masculine traits. Sertoli cells are also known as 'nurse' cells or 'mother cells' or 'sustentacular cells' because they play an important role in the formation of gonadal cells.

Apart from endocrine, sperm production is affected by testicular size, season, nutrition, hormone levels, environmental conditions, and animal health. The duration of spermatogenesis varies greatly between domestic animals (Table 7.5).

Table 7.5: Reference value for the duration of spermatogenesis in domestic animals:

Animals	Bull	Ram	Boar	Stallion	Dog
Spermatogenesis (days)	60-70	60-70	50-60	50-60	50-60

7.7. Semen Evaluation

Semen is a secretory product of the testes and male accessory sex glands that comprises male gametes (spermatozoa) and seminal plasma. Spermatozoa mix with the seminal plasma during emission and ejaculation. The migration of sperm into the pelvic urethra is referred to as emission. The forced release of sperm from the urethra into the penis is referred to as ejaculation.

Seminal plasma is a secretory product of the male accessory sex gland. Male accessory sex glands include the ampullae, the prostrate, the seminal vesicles, and the bulbourethral gland (Cowper's gland). Except for dogs, all domestic species have bulbourethral glands. Vesicular glands are often paired and composed of simple columnar glandular epithelium. These glands are absent in carnivores but present in horses, ruminants, and swine.

The quality of sperm is critical in determining male fertility. Semen analysis is performed to determine male breeding soundness and to select semen samples for artificial insemination (AI), intracytoplasmic sperm injection (ICSI), *in vitro* fertilization (IVF), etc.

Semen analysis (semenalysis) is performed to evaluate the pathophysiology of sperm. A variety of tests are available to evaluate the functional attributes of sperm. So far, no single test has been able to provide information on all sperm characteristics and accurately predict the fertility of a semen sample. As a result, the method used to evaluate semen samples will be determined by the goal of the evaluation and the available resources. The Table 7.6 below shows the minimum requirements for the maximum fertility potential of bull and boar semen samples.

Table 7.6: Minimum standard for probable fertile bull and boar semen:

Parameters	Bull semen	Boar semen
Sperm concentration	Over 500 million sperm per mL.	100 million sperm per mL, with at least 60 to 75 mL produced per ejaculate.
Sperm morphology	Less than 20% of morphological abnormalities.	Less than 20% of morphological abnormalities.
Forward progressive motility	50%	65%

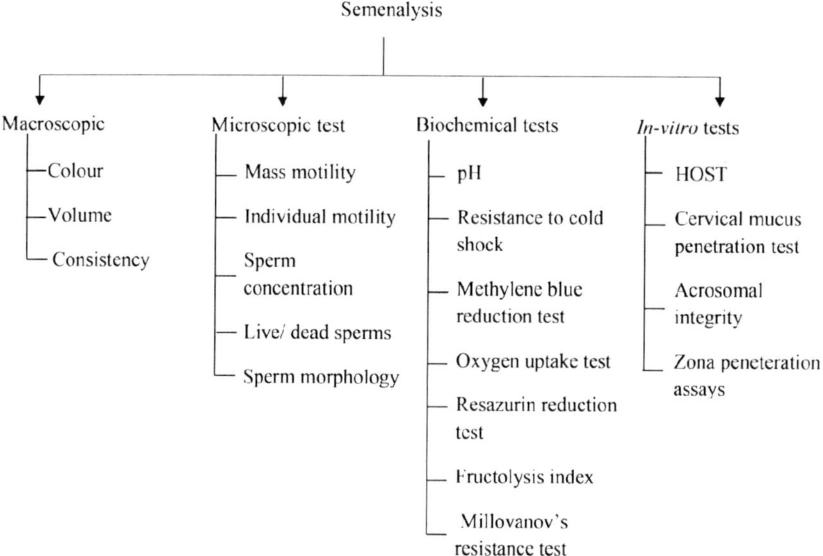

7.8. Macroscopic Examination of Semen

The semen sample has been examined with the naked eye without the use of a microscope. This test must be performed on freshly collected semen samples in order to evaluate sperm characteristics such as volume, colour, consistency, or density. The consistency of most species semen is homogenous. The opacity of semen provides a rough indication of concentration, although it varies from species to species, from ejaculate to ejaculate, and even from individual to individual.

Materials required

- Artificial vagina, graduate semen collection tube, and trained male animal for semen collection.

Procedure

- Collect the semen sample using the artificial vagina method. The other methods of collecting semen from domestic animals include electrical ejaculation, massage, gloved hand, and sponge method.
- Record the volume of semen ejaculated immediately after semen collection by reading the calibrated scale of the graduated semen collection tube (Fig.7.4). Ejaculated semen volume varies from species to species in animals (Table 7.7). It also depends on the function of the

male accessory sex glands and other factors like age, breed, species, and method & frequency of collection.

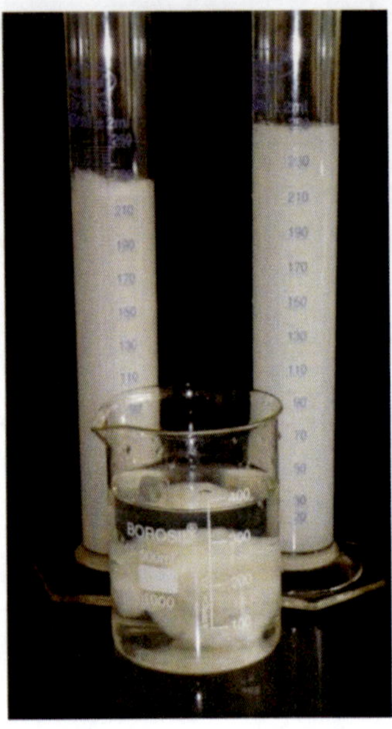

A. Measurement of boar semen and gel mass.

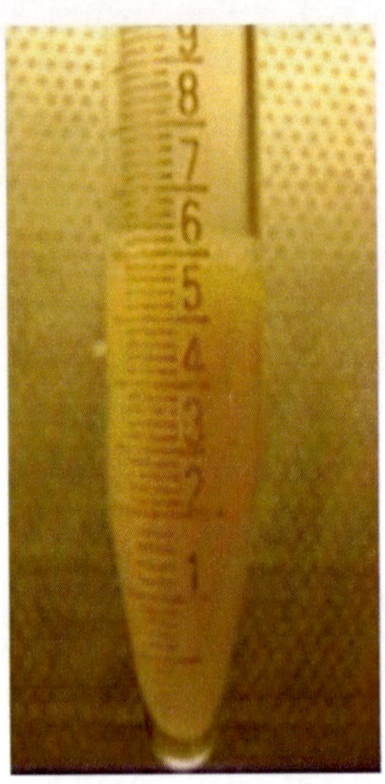

B. Bull semen measurement with a graduated semen collection tube.

Fig. 7.4: Illustration of boar and bull semen volumes

- Then, observe the colour of the semen sample. The normal semen colour varies from species to species in animals (Table 7.8). It is usually milky white or creamy white. A deviation from the normal colour indicates pathological conditions in the genital tract of male animals. For example, blood-stained semen implies genital tract injury. Semen that is yellowish or dark creamish in colour indicates genital tract infection. Orchitis is indicated by the brownish colour of the semen.
- Tilt the semen collection tube containing the semen sample to check the consistency of the semen. Semen consistency is proportional to sperm concentration (Table 7.9) and frequency of collection (Table 7.9).

Table 7.7: Reference values for semen volume in domestic animals:

Sl.No	Animals	Ejaculate volume (mL)	
		Average	Range
1	Bull	4.0	2.0-10.0
2	Buffalo bull	3.0	2.0-80
3	Ram	1.0	0.5-2.0

Sl.No	Animals	Ejaculate volume (mL)	
		Average	Range
4	Buck	1.0	0.5-1.5
5	Boar	250	100-500
6	Stallion	70	30-300
7	Dog	9.0	2-15

Table 7.8: Normal colour of semen in different domestic animals:

Sl No	Animals	Colour
1	Bull	Creamy white
2	Buffalo bull	Milky white
3	Ram	Creamy white
4	Buck	Creamy white
5	Boar	Grayish white
6	Stallion	Grayish white
7	Dog	Milky white

Table 7.9: Assessment of sperm concentrations in rams based on consistency:

Score	Consistency	Number of spermatozoa (X 10^9)	
		Mean	Range
5	Thick creamy	5.0	4.5-6.0
4	Creamy	4.0	3.5-4.5
3	Thin creamy	3.0	2.5-3.5
2	Milky	2.0	1.0-2.5
1	Cloudy	0.7	0.3-1.0
0	Clear / watery	Insignificant	

7.9. Assessment of Sperm Motility

Sperm acquires motility during epididymal transport based on the normal development of axonemes, the presence of mitochondria, and flagellum implantation at the nucleus. This test comprises a subjective assessment of sperm viability and motility quality. Sperm motility patterns are categorized as follows:

A. Mass motility

B. Initial or individual motility

7.9.a. Mass Motility

The collective or wave-like motion of sperm is referred to as mass motility. Mass motility is the first test that determines whether an ejaculate is suitable for further processing or not. In neat semen sample, mass motility is evaluated. However, it is usually assessed in semen samples with a higher sperm concentration per mL, such as ram, buck, or bull semen. The mass mobility of semen samples from dogs, boars, and stallions cannot be assessed.

Materials required

- Neat semen, spirit lamp, pipette, glass slide, slide warmer, phase contrast microscope with Biotherm (37°C), etc.

Procedure

- Put a drop of neat semen on a clean glass slide that has been pre-warmed to 37°C immediately after the collection of the semen.
- Examine the semen drop without a coverslip under a microscope with low-power objective (10x) on a warm Biotherm stage (37°C).
- Observe sperm's movements or their wavelike motion (Fig. 7.5) and assign it a score between 0 and 5, as given in Table 7.10. Only semen samples from fourth and fifth grades are advised for further processing or testing.

Table 7.10: Grading and interpretation of mass motility:

Microscopic appearance	Rating/ numerical scale	Remarks/ Descriptive value
Total immobility	0	All the sperm are dead.
Individual movement	1	Very poor. Motile sperm between ≥ 20 %
Very slow movement	2	Poor. Motile sperm between 20-40 %
General wave movement, slow amplitude of waves	3	Fair. Motile sperm between 60 -80 %
Rapid wave motion, no eddies	4	Good. Motile sperm about 90 %
Rapid wave motion, extremely rapid waves and eddies, about 90-100 % active sperms	5	Excellent. Motile sperm nearly 100%

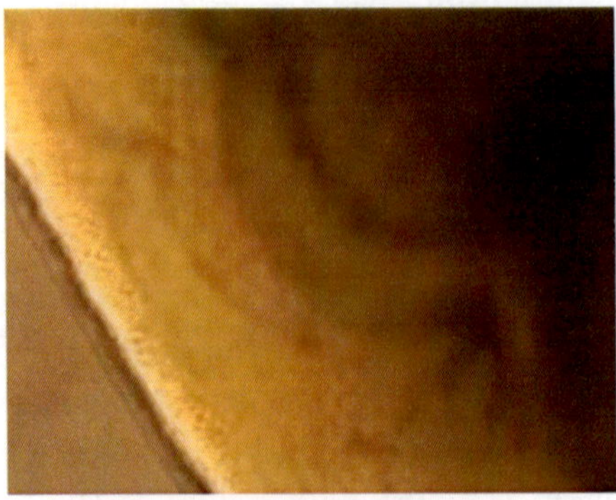

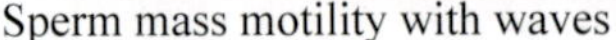

Sperm mass motility with waves

Sperm mass motility without waves

Fig. 7.5: Sperm mass motility

7.9.b. Individual or Initial Motility

The concentration of gradually motile sperm in a semen sample determines its superiority. Weakly motile sperm may generally be senile in cripples. When diluted sperm with an appropriate sperm extender is examined under a microscope, various kinds of distinct individual sperm motility are seen. The following types of sperm motility can be observed, depending on the quality of the sperm:

1. *Progressive motility*- Sperm move in a straight line from one point to another in a progressive and forward motion.
2. *Circular motility*- The movement of sperms with a radius equal to the sperm's length. This movement is seen in associated with sperm defects, especially in the middle piece and tail.
3. *Oscillatory motility*-Side-to-side motion in a static position without change in place. This movement is seen in associated with sperm defects, especially in the middle piece, and tail. It is also seen in associated with aged sperm.
4. *Reverse motility*- Motion in the opposite direction.

Materials required

- Spirit lamp, glass rod, pipette, glass slide, coverslip, slide warmer, phase contrast microscope with Biotherm (37°C).

Reagents

- 2.94 % sodium citrate buffer or tris buffer or tris-egg yolk extender.

Procedure

- Dilute the semen sample (1:100 dilution) with tris buffer, 2.9% sodium citrate buffer (pH 6), or tris-egg yolk extender.
- Put a drop of diluted semen on a clean glass slide that has been preheated to 37°C, and then cover it with a coverslip.
- Examine the glass slide under a microscope with a high-power (40x) objective.
- Observe the initial motility pattern. Count only progressively motile sperm. A good semen sample should have an initial progressive motility of 70% or above.

Table 7.11: Types of sperm motility and their descriptive value

S.No	Progressive motility (%)	Descriptive value
1	≥ 80	Excellent
2	60-80	Good
3	40-60	Fair
4	20-40	Poor
5	0-20	Very poor

Note: The individual or early motility of sperm and their fertility are affected by certain inherited sperm abnormalities, such as diadem, knobbed, decapitated, corkscrew, middle piece, narrow head, etc. Sperm motility is also influenced by the collection method, collection interval, and heat or thermal shock.

7.10. Determination of Spermatozoa Concentration

The test provides information on the quality and concentration of sperm. The total number of spermatozoa in a semen samples is useful in assessing the quality and determining the dilution rate with semen extenders for artificial insemination. There are two methods for determining spermatozoa concentration, which are as follows:

A. Haemocytometer method
B. Photoelectric colorimeter method

7.10.a. Haemocytometer Method

The haemocytometer method is widely used for counting sperm concentration and is regarded the "gold standard" test. In this method, counts sperm directly from diluted spermatozoa under a microscope, then multiplies the result by the dilution factor to get the total number of spermatozoa per mL.

Materials required

- Test tube, pipette, haemocytometer, compound microscope, and semen sample.

Reagents

- Semen diluting fluid: It contains
  - Eosin (water soluble) :0.05 g
  - Sodium chloride :1.0 g
  - Distilled water :100 mL and a drop of formalin.

Procedure

- Mount a haemotocytometer on the microscope stage and focus Nebauer's counting chamber with a low objective (10x) for counting spermatozoa.

- Mix 10 μL of semen with 990 μL diluting fluid (1:100 dilutions).
- Draw a diluted semen sample up to the 0.5 mark of the RBC diluting pipette.
- Clean the tip of the RBC dilution pipette.
- Then, draw the semen-diluting fluid up to 101 mark on the RBC diluting pipette.
- Mix the pipette by rolling it between your palms for 2-3 minutes.
- Discard a few drops of diluted semen and charge the Nebauer's counting chamber of the haemocytometer.
- Wait for 2-3 minutes to allow the spermatozoa to settle down.
- Then, manually count the spermatozoa in 5 secondary squares using a microscope's high-power objective.

Calculation

1.	One primary square has 1 mm length, 1 mm width	
2.	The primary square is divided into 5 X 5	= 25 secondary squares
3.	So, the surface area of one secondary square will be (Length X Width)	$\frac{1}{5} \text{ x } \frac{1}{5} = \frac{1}{25}$ mm^2
4.	The cubic volume of one secondary square will be (surface area X height) So, the cubic volume of five secondary squares will be	$\frac{1}{25}$ mm^2 X $\frac{1}{10}$ mm $= \frac{1}{250} mm^3$ $= 5 \text{ X } \frac{1}{250}$ mm^3 $= \frac{1}{50}$ mm^3
5.	If the blood is taken up to the 0.5 mark in the RBC pipette, then the dilution factorwill be	= 200
6.	Let us assume the total number of cells counted in the 5 secondary squares (80 small squares) is "X" in mm^3 of blood	
7.	Therefore, the number of spermatozoa present in 1mm^3 of diluted blood will be	$= 50 \times X$
8.	Now, it can be said that $50 \times X$ number of spermatozoa are present in 1 mm^3 volumeof undiluted semen	
9.	Here, as semen is diluted (1:100) and dilution factoris 200. so No. of spermatozoa present in examined diluted semen is	$= 50 \times X \times 100X\ 200/mm^3$ $=X \times 10^6/mm^3$

The number of spermatozoa present in the semen sample is expressed as million/μL or cmm.

7.10.b. Photoelectric Colorimeter Method

In this method, the concentration of sperm is determined based on Beer-Lambert's Law. The optical density (OD) or absorbance of the semen sample is proportional to its concentration. Hence, the sperm concentration is determined from a standard curve by plotting OD on the Y-axis against the known sperm concentration on the X-axis.

Materials required

- Test tube, pipette, spectrophotometer, haemocytometer, and semen sample.

Reagents

- Semen diluting fluid- It contains

a. Eosin (water soluble) :0.05 g

b. Sodium chloride :1.0 g

c. Distilled water :100 mL and a drop of formalin

Procedure

- Dilute the semen sample with a 3% sodium citrate solution as follows:

Sl No	Semen (mL)	Sodium citrate (mL)
1	0.1	9.9
2	0.2	9.8
3	0.3	9.7
4	0.4	9.6
5	0.5	9.5
6	0.6	9.4
7	0.7	9.3
8	0.8	9.2
9	0.9	9.1
10	1.0	9.0

- Determine the total spermatozoa for each dilution as per the aforementioned haemocytometer method.
- Read the OD for each serial dilution at 620nm wavelength in a spectrophotometer.
- Draw a standard curve by plotting OD at the Y axis versus sperm concentration at the X axis.

- Then dilute the unknown semen sample (0.2 mL) with 3% sodium citrate (9.8 mL), read the OD at 620nm, and calculate the spermatozoa concentration from the standard curve.

Sperm Concentrations in Domestic animals

Animal species have different spermatozoa concentrations. (Table7.12). Additionally, it varies with age, testicular size, extragonadal sperm reserve size, season, frequency of ejaculation, and various reproductive diseases.

Table 7.12: Reference values for spermatozoa concentration in domestic animals:

Sl No	Animals	Spermatozoa concentration (10^6/mL)	
		Range	Average
1	Bull	300-2000	1000
2	Buffalo bull	200-800	600
3	Ram	2000-6000	3000
4	Buck	1000-5000	3000
5	Stallion	30-800	120
6	Boar	25-300	100
7	Dog	60-300	300
8	Cat	100-2600	1700

Oligozoospermia

- Virus infection
- Hormonal imbalance
- Testicular hypoplasia
- Ttesticular degeneration

Polyzoospermia

- Polyzoosperima cases are reared in animals

7.11. Live and Dead Sperm Count

The test is based on the idea that eosin stains only dead sperm and turns them dark pink due to its enhanced permeability within the cell membrane. Nigrosin increases the contrast between the background and the sperm heads, making it easier to distinguish between sperm under a microscope.

Materials required

- Watch glass, glass slide, pipette, hot plate, glass beaker, phase contrast microscope and semen sample.

Reagents

- Eosin and nigrosin stain: Dissolve 0.67 g of eosin-Y and 0.9 g of sodium chloride in 100 mL of distilled water in a glass beaker placed on a stirring hot plate. Then add 10.0 g of nigrosin, after a gentle heating of the solution.

Procedure

- Mix 50µL of eosin–nigrosin stain with 50µL diluted semen in a microtube.
- Hold at 37^{0}C at least for 30 seconds.
- Prepare a thin smear on a grease-free glass slide and dry it.
- Count the number of live and dead spermatozoa in the smear using a phase contrast microscope's oil immersion objective (100x). Live spermatozoa are not stained, whereas dead spermatozoa are coloured pink (Fig.7.6).
- Count at least 200 different spermatozoa in different fields. Count separately for live and dead spermatozoa.
- Calculate the percentage of live and dead spermatozoa as shown below.

$$\text{Live spermatozoa (\%)} = \frac{\text{Numbers of live spermatozoa counted}}{\text{Total number of spermatozoa counted}} \text{ X } 100$$

$$\text{Dead spermatozoa (\%)} = \frac{\text{Numbers of dead spermatozoa counted}}{\text{Total number of spermatozoa counted}} \text{ X } 100$$

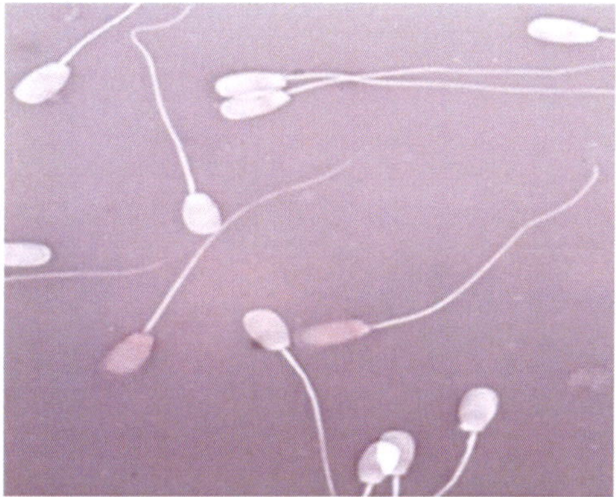

Fig. 7.6: Eosin and nigrosin staining. Live spermatozoa are unstained; dead spermatozoa are stained pink or red.

7.12. Sperm Morphology and Counting of Abnormal Sperm

The morphology of most mammalian species sperm is almost 50 μM in length. Round spermatids evolve into spermatids with varying degrees of elongation, and then into spermatozoa. Mammalian sperm is divided into three different parts: the head, middle piece, and tail. The oval-shaped head contains haploid DNA and the acrosome. The acrosome is derived from the Golgi apparatus and contains enzymes like acrosin, hyaluronidase, proacrosin, esterase, phospholipase A_2, acid phosphatases, aryl-sulphatase, -N-acetyl glucosaminidase, aryl-amidase, and non-specific acid proteinases that differ quantitatively or qualitatively among species. Hyaluronidase and aryl-sulphatase aid sperm penetration through the cumulus oophorus.The axoneme is the central core of sperm that extends from the base of the head to the entire length of the tail. The axonemes in the centre are surrounded by mitochondria, which provide energy in the form of ATP for sperm survival and movement.

Any deviation in the morphology of sperm from normal is regarded as abnormal. Morphological abnormalities are often found in the head, neck, middle piece, and tail (Table 7.13 and Fig.7.6). Sperm abnormalities have been classified as primary, secondary, and tertiary. Primary abnormalities are deformities of the sperm that develop during spermatogenesis. It may be due to defects in the seminiferous tubules and caput of the epididymis. Secondary abnormalities arise during the maturation of sperm. Human intervention causes tertiary abnormalities. It originates during laboratory handling and processing of the semen sample.

Table 7.13: Different types of sperm abnormalities:

Abnormality	Head	Neck	Middle piece	Tail
i) Primary	a) Mega head. b) Micro head. c) Taping head. d) Pyriform head. e) Double head. f) Swollen head. g) Ghost head.	a) Asymmetrical neck. b) Abaxial neck. c) Broken neck.	a) Absence of mid piece. b) Sheath less midpiece.	a) Tailless. b) Shorter tail.
ii) Secondary	a) Burst head. b) Swollen head. c) Degeneration of sheath in the head.	a) Broken neck.	a) Swollen mid piece.	a) Coiled tail.
iii) Tertiary	------------	--------	a) Broken mid piece.	a) Coiled tail. b) Bent tail. c) Loop tail. d) Tail bent over the head. e) Tail bent over the head at 180^0.

Morphologic abnormalities have a significant impact on fertility. This is why; the evaluation of sperm morphology is an integral part of routine semen analysis. The morphology of sperm is studied under a microscope using an eosin-nigrosin or toluidine stain. Sperm are clearly visible after staining when seen with an oil immersion objective (100x). The percentage of sperm abnormalities can be calculated by counting 200 spermatozoa in different fields.

Materials required

- Watch glass, glass slide, pipette, phase contrast microscope, thermostat and semen sample.

Reagents

- 3% sodium citrate: Dissolve 3 g of sodium citrate in distilled water and make the volume 100 mL.
- Rose bengal stain: Dissolve 3 g of rose Bengal in distilled water, add 1 mL of formalin, and finally make the volume 100 mL with distilled water.

Procedure

- Mix one drop of semen with 10 drops of 3% sodium citrate solution at 37°C in a watch glass.
- Prepare a smear of the diluted semen sample on a grease-free glass slide and dry it.
- Then stain it with Rose Bengal stain for 15 minutes.
- Dip the slide into distilled water to remove the excess stain.
- Dry the smear and observe it under a microscope with low and high power objectives.
- Observe at least 200 spermatozoa on a stained slide at random. It is preferable to count the abnormal spermatozoa on two distinct slides.

Note*:* In animals, every ejaculation contains between 5 to15% abnormal sperm. AI is not advised for semen samples with more than 20% morphological abnormalities.

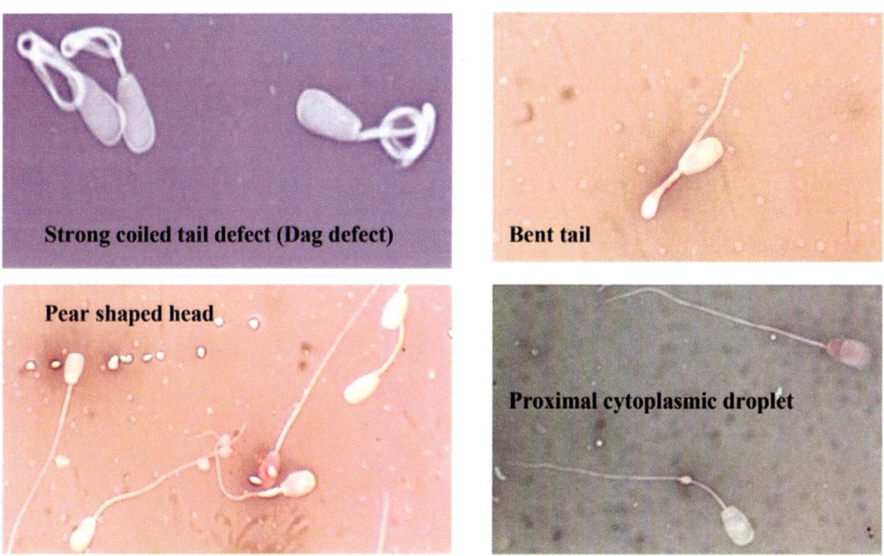

Fig. 7.7: Illustration of morphological abnormalities in sperm

7.13 Nomenclature use in semen analysis

Semen Parameter	Evaluation criteria	Nomenclature
Volume	None	Aspermia
	Reduced	Hypospermia
	Increased	Hyperspermia
Sperm concentration	Zero	Azoospermia
	Reduced	Oligozoospermia
	Normal	Normo-zoospermia
Sperm motility	Decreased	Astheno-zoospermia
Sperm viability	All dead	Necrozoospermia
Abnormal sperm	High percentage	Terato-zoospermia
Sperm shape	Only round headed sperms	Globospermia
Abnormal semen	Blood or pus in semen	Hemospermia or pyospermia

8

Animal Growth and Surface Area Measurement

8.0. Introduction

Growth is the irreversible gain in body weight, size, length, and circumference. It is accomplished by two fundamental processes: hypertrophy (increase in tissue, cell volume and progressive accumulation of intercellular substances) and hyperplasia (growth as a result of cellular multiplication by mitotic division). Animal growth is influenced by both genetic and environmental factors.

Animal body growth and weight gain play a critical role in reproductive performance. It also acts as one of the traits to evaluate the breeding value, optimize management & feeding practices, and prepare the correct dose of therapeutic pharmaceuticals to treat animal diseases. As a result, measurement of body growth is essential for the selection of superior germplasm, feeding & housing management, health care management, and optimizing other environmental conditions that have an impact on animal growth for an economically viable animal industry.

8.1. Measurement of Prenatal Growth

Prenatal growth (from conception to birth) and postnatal growth (from birth till old age) are the two distinct stages of animal growth. During the prenatal phase, the fetus actual weight is very difficult to determine. In general, the fetal size is judged based on fetometric measurements, which are illustrated in Fig. 8.1.

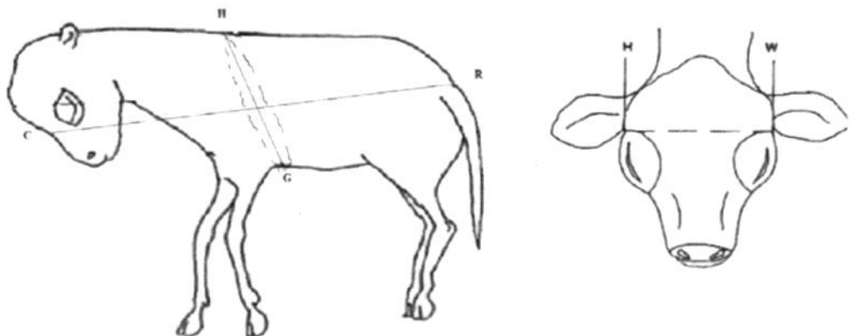

Fig. 8.1: Illustration of reference points for measurements of prenatal growth in animals.

Fetometric measurements are

1. Crown-Rump-Length (CRL): It gives the length of the fetus. It is measured from the top of the head, or crown to the bottom of the buttocks, or rump, as illustrated in Fig.8.1.
2. Heart Girth (GH) or Trunk diameter: It is measured at the widest point in the region of the last ribs, at the level of the liver and stomach, as illustrated in Fig.8.1.
3. Head Width (HW): It is measured at the widest distance between the zygomatic arches in the head, as illustrated in Fig.8.1.

Based on the above measurements (Fig.8.1), the prenatal growth of animals is measured or judged with the help of the following tools:

1. Ultrasonography
2. X-ray
3. Computerized Tomography Scan (CT scan)
4. Magnetic Resonance Imagination (MRI)

Real-time B-mode diagnostic scanners have been widely used in animal reproduction as well as the judgment of fetal growth. The Table 8.1 below shows the relationship between CRL and the body weight of the bovine fetus.

Table 8.1: Average CRL of bovine fetus at different ages and their corresponding body weight:

Age (days)	CR length (in cm)	Weight of the fetus
30	1	0.5g
60	5	5.9g
90	13	72.6g
120	30	531g
150	38	1.6 kg
180	56	3.8 kg
210	71	9.5 kg
245	81	17.7 kg
280	86	28.6 kg

Note: The process of prenatal growth is complex. Both the genetics of the fetus and environmental factors influence prenatal growth. Environmental factors include maternal factors (maternal nutrition, parity, lactation, physiological status of the mother, and gestation length), and ambient temperature, etc.

8.2. Measurement of Postnatal Growth

The postnatal growth rate of animals is calculated using different growth rates and growth curves, based on body weight and age.

1. Absolute growth rate

It is defined as absolute gain in weight per unit of time. The absolute weight gain per unit time = $(W_2 - W_1) / (t_2 - t_1)$

Where, W_1 = Initial weight, W_2= Final weight and $(t_2 - t_1)$ = Time interval between two measurements.

2. Relative growth rate

It is defined as the weight gained in a specific time in relation to the weight at the beginning of that time. It is expressed in percentage.

So, relative growth rate (%) = $(W_2 - W_1) / (W_1 x100)$

Where

W_1 = Initial weight, W_2= Final weight.

3. Specific or Instantaneous growth rate

It is the logarithm of size or weight plotted against the age of the animal.

Instantaneous growth rate = (dw/dt)/W

Where, dw/dt is the instantaneous weight gain and W is the initial weight. Practically, it is impossible to measure the instantaneous weight gain.

So, it can be calculated by following the formula:

$K = (\ln W_2 - \ln W_1)/ t_2 - t_1$

Where,

ln: Natural logarithm.

W_2 & W_1: Final and initial body weights, respectively.

t_1 & t_2: Initial and final recorded time, respectively.

Time required to double the body weight = $\ln_2/K$.

8.3. Growth curve

The growth curve describes how an animal's body size or mass changes over time. It is most often used to illustrate animal growth trends and to predict the expected weight of animals at a specific age. The growth curve has two different phases: the accelerating phase and the decelerating phase, or retarding phase and it is "S"-shaped or sigmoid in shape. The growth curve is prepared by plotting the weight of an animal against its age. The live weight of animals is widely used to determine the postnatal growth of animals.

Methods of body weight measurement

a. Direct method

b. Indirect method

8.3.a. Direct method

The body weight of animals is measured with a weighbridge. In this method, animals are allowed to stand on a weighbridge platform for 10 to 15 seconds before recording their weight on the scale in kg. This method can also be used to track how an animal's weight increases with age by measuring the animal's weight at different intervals.

8.3.b. Indirect method

In this method, the live body weight of an animal is calculated with the help of a formula based on the following body measurements, as shown in Fig. 8.2. A measuring tape is used to take the body measurements.

- Body Height (BH): It is measured from the floor to the highest point of the withers (i.e., the highest part of the vertebral column of the animal between the shoulder blades), as shown in Fig.8.2.
- Body length (BL): It is measured from the point of shoulder to the point of pin bone, as shown in Fig. 8.2.
- Heart Girth (HG): The circumference of the body over the chest of the animal is just behind the point of the elbow, as shown in Fig. 8.2.

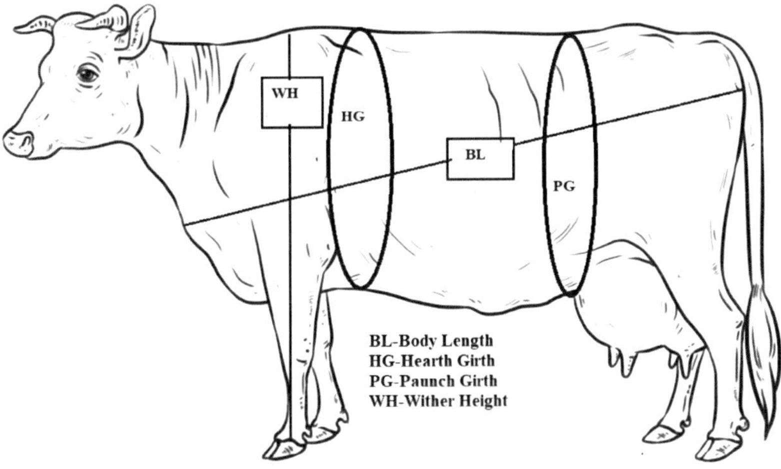

Fig. 8.2: Illustration of reference points for body measurements

- Calculate the body weight of animals using the following formula below.

1. Shaffer's formula

Weight in pounds (Ib) $\text{Weight} = \frac{(\text{G in inches x L in inches})}{Y}$

Where, L = Body length in inches and G = Heart Girth in inches.

2. Aggarwal's formula

It is the modified Shaeffer's formula developed for the Indian cattle.

$$\text{Weight} = \frac{(\text{G in inches x L in inches})}{\text{Y}}$$

Where, Y = 9.0 if the girth is less than 65 inches, Y = 8.5 if it is between 65 and 80 inches, and Y =8.0 if it is over 80 inches.

8.4. Measurement of Body Surface Area

The skin that covers an animal's body surface serves as a feedforward signal for the thermoregulatory system for heat exchange mechanisms *via* conduction, convection, and radiation, in addition to acting as a protective barrier between internal and external environments, particularly in the tropics. The body surface area of animals can be accurately measured using a device known as a "**surface integrator**". This technique is based on the rolling of a revolving metal cylinder with a known area that is attached to a revolution counter. The surface area is calculated by multiplying the number of revolutions by the area of the roller.

Materials required

- Surface integrator, measuring tape and white chalk, etc.
- *Surface integrator*: There are two wheels on the device. The wheel is connected to a revolution counter. The other wheel is connected with white chalk in such a way that it leaves a white line on the surface over which it runs. The following formula is used to calculate the area covered.

A = (Circumference of the wheel) X (Distance between two wheels) X (Number of revolutions)

Where, A = Area in cm^2

Procedure

- Measure the surface area for the trunk, legs, tail, head, and ear; preferably, the animal is standing on all four legs, as per the procedure mentioned below.
- The total body surface area (in cm^2) is calculated by the following equation.

  Body surface area= 2 (M + F + R + E) + T + H

  Where,

  M is the area of trunk

  F is the area of the fore leg

  R is the area of the rear leg

  E is the area of the ear

  T is the area of the tail

  H is the area of the head

Procedure for measurement of the surface area of the trunk (M)

- Measure the surface area of one side of an animal as shown in Fig.8.3 with a surface integrator.
- Set the surface integrator's counter to zero (zero), and then push it from the base of the tail up to the shoulder along the spinal column's midline.
- When the integrator reaches the shoulder, lift it off.
- Continue until the midline of the chest and belly is fully reached.

- Read the counter and note it.
- The surface integrator's counter is reset to zero, and then run over the area between the shoulder and head in vertical strips from the lower midline to the centre of the spinal column. At the time of measurement the animal's head is turned in the opposite direction to remove the wrinkles in the skin and the hand is held on opposite side of the dewlap.
- Read the counter and note it. Calculate the area using the following formula.

  Area= Circumference x length

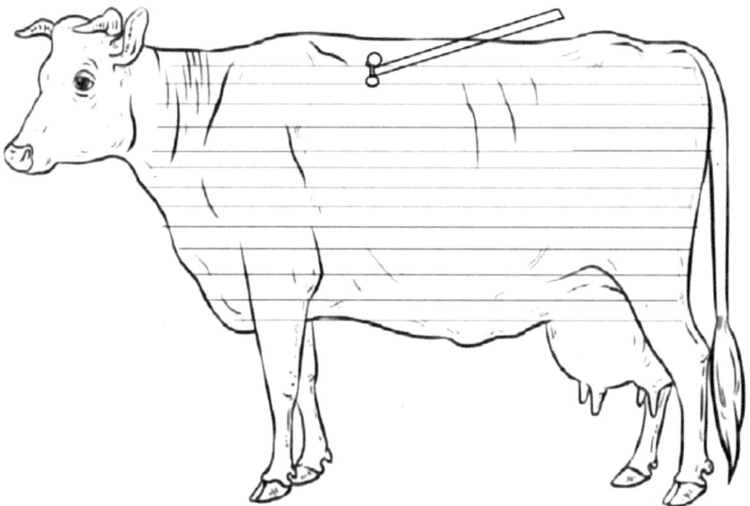

Fig. 8.3: Measurement of the surface area by surface integrator

Procedure for measurement of the surface area of the legs

- Measure the area of the fore (F) and hind (R) legs with the integrator by placing the legs wide apart. Run the integrator around the legs down to the vicinity of the knee and hock joints.
- Then, measure the length from the last mark of the integrator to the top of the hoof for the lower part of the legs below the hock and knee joint.
- Measure the circumferences first just below the last line of the integrator, the second and third just above and below the middle of the shank; and the fourth at the pastern. Then calculate the area separately for F and R.

Procedure for measurement of the surface area of a tail (T)

- Measure the length of the tail from the base to the tip of the last coccygeal vertebrae.
- Measure five circumferences at different places, viz., first at the base, second and fourth just above and below the middle of the tail, third at the middle, and fifth just above the switch. Then, calculate the average circumference.
- Calculate the area using the following formula.

  Area = Circumference x length

Procedure for measurement of the surface area of a head (H)

- Measure the length of the head from the top of the poll to the tip of the mouth. Likewise, measure the width from the base of one ear to the other.
- Calculate the area using the following formula.

  Area = ½ width x length

Procedure for measurement of the surface area of the ear (E)

- Measure the outside longitudinal length of the ear from the base to the tip.
- Measure the circumference of the flattened ear at the middle of its length, where it is widest.
- Calculate the area using the following formula.

  Area = Width x length

Note: The body surface area of an animal is a good indicator of how well it can withstand or adapt a hot climate.

8.5. Growth Regulator

There are numerous chemicals that have a significant impact on growth. These chemicals are classified 1. Tissue-specific growth factor 2. Hormonal systems 3. Feed additives and other substances. Tissue-specific growth factors influence cellular growth regulators by regulating the proliferation and development of specific types of cells.

Table 8.2: Tissue-specific growth factors

S.No.	Growth factors	Effects
1	Epidermal growth factor	Stimulate cell proliferation both *in vivo* and *in vitro.*
2	Nerve growth factor	Regulates the growth, maintenance, and development of sympathetic and embryonic sensory neurons.
3	Erythropoietin	Stimulate the production of red blood cells. It promotes the synthesis of RNA, haemoglobin, and numerous enzymes in erythroid cells.
4	Promine and Retine	Promine is a growth promoter. Retine acts as a growth inhibitor.
5	Chalones	Chalone suppresses the mitotic activity of the tissue in which it is produced.

9

Environmental Physiology Meteorological Variables and Health Parameters

9.0. Introduction

Climate change induces significant and long-lasting shifts in the statistical distribution of weather patterns over periods ranging from decades to million years. It is believed to be the cause of long-term temperature changes, changes in rainfall patterns and volume, prolonged summer seasons, increasing sea levels, and increased frequency and intensity of floods, droughts, and heat waves, etc.

Animals are intimately and inseparately associated with their physiological and chemical environments from conception until death. As a result, climate change has an impact on animals both directly and indirectly. Since, animals have had to alter their behavioural and physiological mechanisms in order to maintain homeostasis.

Climate change has emerged as a serious threat to the livestock industry. It reduces animal productivity by lowering growth, milk yield, meat production, egg production, wool production, reproductive performance, and health. About 20 to 30 percent of plant and animal species would likely be at risk of extinction with an increase of 1.5 to 2.5°C, which will result in severe consequences for food and nutritional security in developing countries. This is why; measurements of meteorological variables are needed for effective scientific management of livestock and poultry to cope with the negative impacts of climate change while enhancing growth and productivity.

9.1. Measurement of Ambient Temperature

The term "ambient temperature" simply refers to "the temperature of the surroundings" or the temperature of the immediate surroundings. The intensity or severity of the ambient temperature changes throughout the day;

it is colder at night and warmer during the day. Ambient or air temperature has an impact on domestic animals' productivity and health, both directly and indirectly. Hence, it is essential to provide a thermoneutral zone (TNZ) for farm animals in order to achieve optimum performance and maintain good health. Thermoneutral zone or often known as the comfort zone, is the range of indoor humidity, temperature, and air movement under which an animal feels mental and physical well-being.

In domestic animals, TNZ varies with species (Table 9.1). It also depends on age, breed, species, feed intake, diet composition, the previous state of temperature acclimation or acclimatization, production, specific housing and pen conditions, tissue insulation like fat & skin, external insulation (coat), and the behaviour of the animal, etc. TNZ is bounded by the lower critical temperature (LCT) and upper critical temperature (UCT). UCT is the highest tolerable temperature beyond which serious problems are likely. LCT is defined as the temperature below which a resting animal must increase its metabolic rate from the basal level to meet the environmental demands for heat.

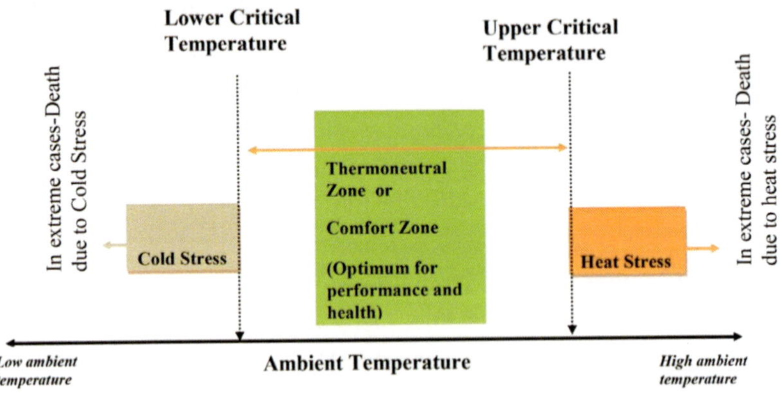

Fig. 9.1: Schematic representation showing the relationship between thermal zones and ambient temperature.

Table 9.1: Thermoneutral or comfort zone of various domestic animals:

S.No	Animals	Thermo-neutral zone
1	Holstein Friesian	5-21°C
2	Jersey and Brown Swiss	5-24°C
3	Crossbred cow (India)	15-25°C
4	Buffalo (India)	13-24°C
5	Adult pigs	18-22 °C

Ambient temperature is measured using thermometers. Most thermometers are in the form of a narrow closed glass tube with an expanded bulb at one end.

Ambient temperature is measured using the following thermometers:

a) Alcohol thermometer

b) Maximum–minimum thermometer

c) Wide range thermometer

d) Long range thermometer

e) Dry and Wet bulb thermometer

f) Infra red thermometer

Celsius (0^0C) and fahrenheit (^{0}F) are the two most commonly used scales in thermometers.

9.1.a. Alcohols thermometer

The alcohol thermometer is an alternative to the mercury-in-glass thermometer (Fig.9.2). Temperatures range from -40°C to 50°C on the Celsius scale and from -40°F to 120°F on the Fahrenheit scale. The alcohol in the bulb rises as the temperature rises, and the temperature is recorded according to the gradation of the thermometer and expressed in ^{0}C and ^{0}F.

Alcohol thermometer is used to monitor the temperature of animal and poultry houses as well as experimental rooms. This thermometer automatically records the ambient temperature.

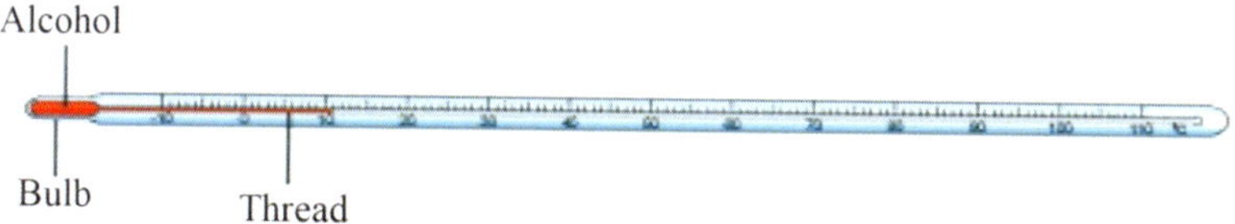

Fig. 9.2: Alcohol thermometer

9.1.b. Maximum and minimum thermometer

Maximum and minimum thermometer contains two glass columns; the left one is for measuring minimum temperature, while the right one is for maximum temperature. The temperature range for both columns is (-) 30°C to 60°C and (-) 20°F to 140°F.

Maximum and minimum thermometer is used to measure the highest (T max) and minimum temperature (T min) of a specified area for a specific time in degrees Celsius or Fahrenheit. The maximum and minimum air temperatures are recorded for the 24 hours, commencing at midnight.

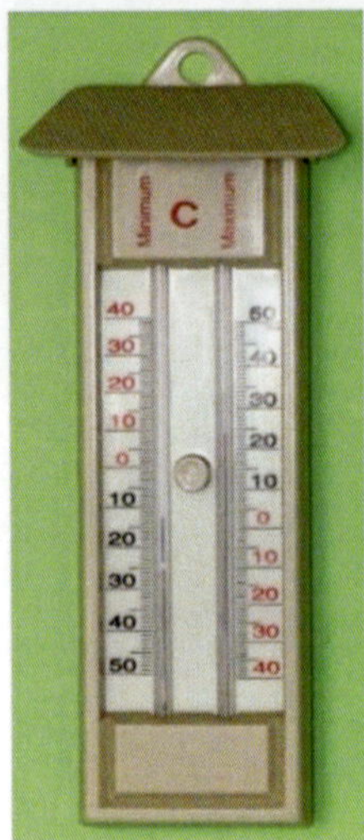

Fig. 9.3: Maximum and minimum thermometer

9.1.c. Wide range thermometer

Wide range thermometer is used for measuring the temperature below 0^0C. The basic characteristics of a wide range thermometer are as follows:

a) It can measure temperature from (-) 30 ^{0}C to 50^0C.

b) Mercury is used as the thermometric fluid.

c) Sub-zero temperature can be measured.

d) It has a prominent safety valve at the head.

e) Nitrogen (N_2 gas) is used as a filling gas.

9.1.d. Long range thermometer

Long range thermometer is used for measuring the melting and boiling temperatures of substances. The basic characteristics of this thermometer are as follows:

a) The temperature ranges from (a) (-) 10^0C to 110^0C or, (b) 0^0C to 200^0C.

b) Broad marking in every 5^0C.

c) Mercury is used as the thermometric fluid.

9.2. Measurement of Humidity

The atmosphere always contains moisture, either in the form of invisible vapours or clouds. The amount of water vapour in the air is measured as humidity. When the air contains lots of water, the weather is described as humid. The most widely employed measurements for atmospheric humidity are absolute and relative humidity. Absolute humidity indicates the moisture content of the atmospheric air and is expressed in either gram per cubic meter (g.m-3) or grams per kilogram (g.kg-1). The relative humidity indicates the present state of absolute humidity relative to the maximum humidity given the same temperature and is normally expressed as a percentage.

9.2.a. Hair hygrometer

Hair hygrometer is a simple instrument to measure the water content of the atmosphere (Fig. 9.4) that can measure the humidity at any given time. The length of the hair expands or shrinks in response to the relative humidity of the atmosphere. The hygrometer ranges from 0% to 100%, with a normal comfort zone marked from 40% to 0%.

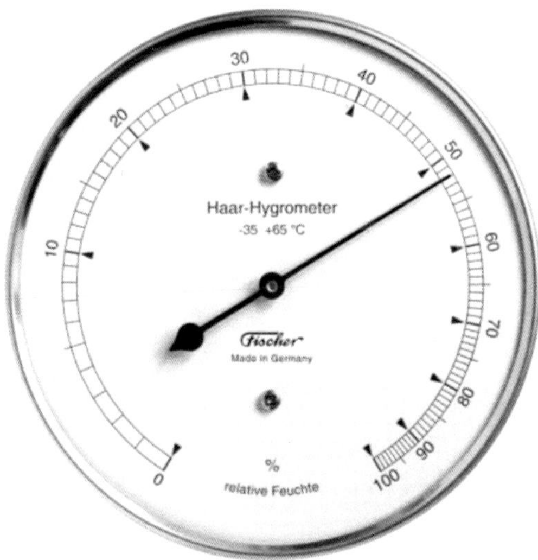

Fig. 9.4: Hair Hygrometer

9.2.b. Dry and wet bulb thermometer

The thermometer is made up of two similar thermometers, namely dry and wet bulb thermometers filled with either mercury or alcohol. The Fahrenheit scale has markings ranging from ranges from 20°F to 120°F. The wet bulb is covered with a fine muslin cloth and is connected by a wick to water held in a small container below. As water evaporates from the muslin cloth, the wet bulb is cooled, and the thermometer gives a lower reading. The air temperature is measured using a dry bulb thermometer. The difference in temperature between the Dry and Wet bulbs is known as Wet-bulb depression, and it is used to calculate air humidity. Dry bulb and wet bulb temperatures can be used directly to calculate relative humidity using a psychrometric chart (Fig 9.5) or a hygrometric table (Table 9.2).

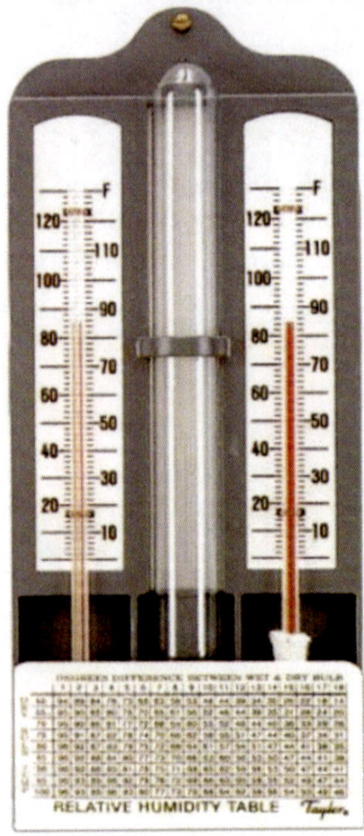

Fig. 9.5: Dry and wet bulb thermometer

9.2.c. Sling psychrometer

Sling psychrometer is used for the instant measurement of relative humidity of an area. The instrument is made up of two mercury thermometers clamped in a frame and attached to a swivel handle, as shown below in Fig. 9.6. The Celsius thermometer has markings ranging from 0°C to 50°C. The wet bulb is wrapped with a cotton cloth. The instrument contains a rotator, which is used to spin the thermometer in order to detect humidity. The relative humidity and vapour pressure can be read directly from the psychometric chart (Fig.9.8).

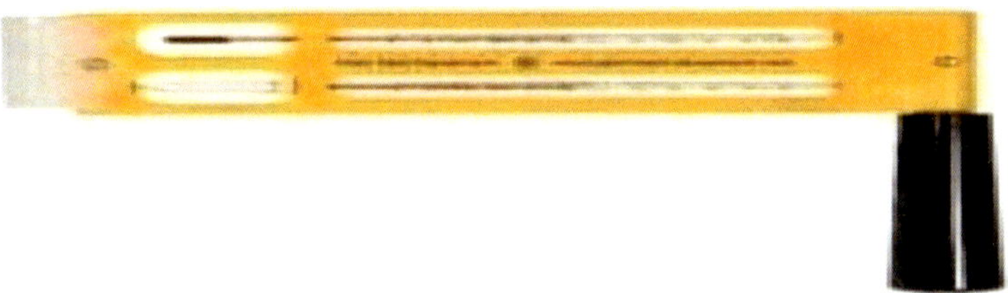

Fig. 9.6: Sling psychrometer

9.2.d. Thermohygrometer (dial type)

A thermohygrometer is an instrument that measures both temperature and humidity at the same time. As shown in Fig. 9.7, the instrument contains two scales: one for humidity and another for temperature. The red scale indicates temperatures from 0 to 40°C. The blue scale indicates the relative humidity from 20 to 100 %, with divisions for each 20%. There are two triangles, one for temperature and one for humidity, indicating the comfort zone.

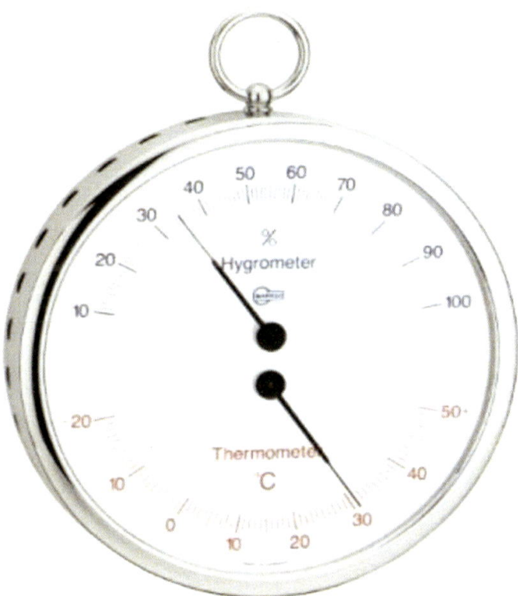

Fig. 9.7: Thermohygrometer

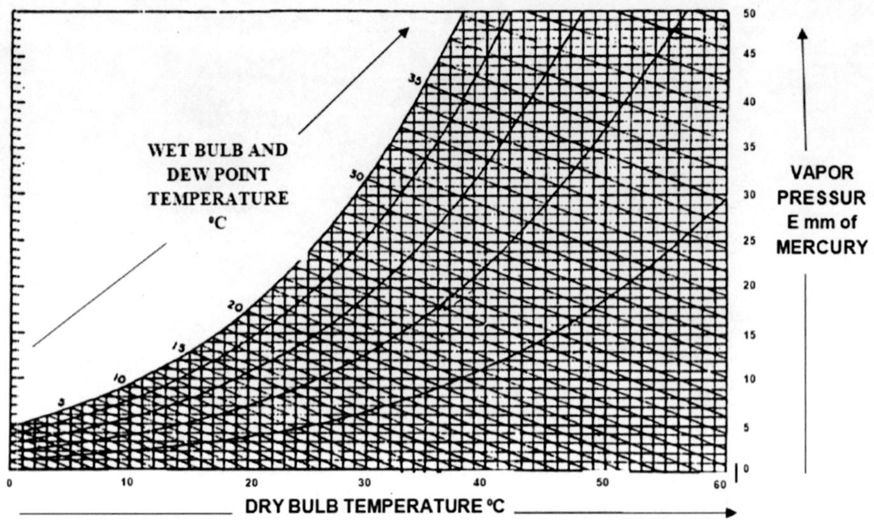

Fig. 9.8: Psychometric chart

Table 9.2: Psychrometric table showing percent relative humidity:

Dry bulb °C	Relative humidity (%)Wet bulb °C									
	28.0	**28.2**	**28.4**	**28.6**	**28.8**	**29.0**	**29.2**	**29.4**	**29.6**	**29.8**
32.0	73	74	75	76	78	79	80	82	83	84
32.2	71	73	74	75	77	78	79	80	82	83
32.4	70	71	73	74	75	77	78	79	81	82
32.6	69	70	72	73	74	75	77	78	79	81
32.8	68	69	70	72	73	74	75	77	78	79
33.0	67	68	69	70	72	73	74	75	77	78
33.2	66	67	68	69	71	72	73	74	76	77
33.4	65	66	67	68	70	71	72	73	74	76
33.6	64	65	66	67	69	70	71	72	73	75
33.8	63	64	65	66	67	69	70	71	72	73
34.0	62	63	64	65	66	67	69	70	71	72
34.2	61	62	63	64	65	66	67	69	70	71
34.4	60	61	62	63	64	65	67	68	69	70
34.6	59	60	61	62	63	64	65	67	68	69
34.8	58	59	60	61	62	63	65	66	67	68
35.0	57	58	59	60	61	62	63	65	66	67
35.2	56	57	58	59	60	61	62	64	65	66
35.4	55	56	57	58	59	60	61	63	64	65
35.6	54	55	56	57	58	59	61	62	63	64
35.8	53	54	55	56	58	59	60	61	62	63

Dry bulb °C	Relative humidity (%)Wet bulb °C									
	28.0	28.2	28.4	28.6	28.8	29.0	29.2	29.4	29.6	29.8
36.0	53	53	54	55	57	58	59	60	61	62
36.2	52	53	54	55	56	57	58	59	60	61
36.4	51	52	53	54	55	56	57	58	59	60
36.6	50	51	52	53	54	55	56	57	58	59
36.8	49	50	51	52	53	54	55	56	57	58
37.0	48	49	50	51	52	53	54	55	56	57
37.2	48	49	49	51	51	53	53	55	55	57
37.4	47	48	49	50	51	52	53	54	55	56
37.6	46	47	48	49	50	51	52	53	54	55
37.8	45	46	47	48	49	50	51	52	53	54

9.2.f. Lambrecht Hygrometer

The Lambrecht hygrometer can constantly record humidity for 24 hours at 15-minute intervals. It has two scales: one for relative humidity (from 0 to 100% with 5% divisions) and one for temperature (from 0 to 50°C). This instrument also has a pointer with ink, which is attached to a horse hair strings. The printer displays the relative humidity percentage on the relative humidity scale based on moisture absorbed from the environment.

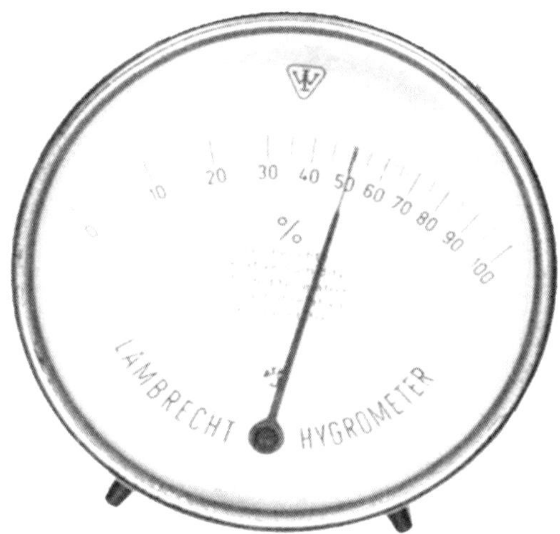

Fig. 9.9: Lambrecht hygrometer

9.3. Temperature Humidity Index

The Temperature Humidity Index (THI) is used to assess the degree of discomfort experienced by animals in hot weather. Johnson (1963) developed this method, which takes into account environmental parameters rather than physiological responses. THI incorporates the effects of both ambient temperature and relative humidity. It is the most basic and practical index for assessing environmental temperature in relation to quantifying heat load on animals, as well as an indicator of stressful thermal climatic conditions. THI is calculated using the following formulas based on dry and wet bulb temperatures:

THI = 0.72 (Dbt + Wbt) + 40.6

Where, Dbt = Dry bulb temperature in °C; Wbt = Wet bulb temperature in °C.

THI = 0.8DBT+ RH x (DBT-14.4) + 46.4

Where, DBT is Dry bulb temperature (°C) and RH is relative humidity.

Interpretation

THI is the most practical and effective way for assessing heat stress in domestic animals.

THI value is

<72= No discomfort or little discomfort.

72-75 =Mild stress.

>75 = Stressful (Feed intake decreases and milk production decreases)

78 -80 = Severe stress.

9.4. Measurement of Wind Direction and Wind Velocity

Wind refers to the movement of air. Wind direction and velocity have a direct impact on the heat exchange mechanism or thermoregulation of animals, and consequently on their growth and metabolism. The direction of wind flow is usually determined by a 'Wind Vane' and the wind velocity is measured by an 'Anemometer'.

9.4.a. Direction of wind flow

The direction of wind flow is usually determined by a 'Wind Vane'. The instrument consists of a pointer with one end arrow-headed (pointing in the windward direction) and the other end termed SAIL (fang) facing the leeward side. The pointer is connected to the central axis, which is fixed to the spindle of a ball-bearing system, allowing the pointer to move in a horizontal plane to show wind direction. Also, there are four cross arms fastened rigidly a bit below the vane and pointing east, south, west, and north. The vane should be mounted at a good height on the top of the vertical post in areas where air passage is not obstructed. The wind vane moves in response to a slight breeze and always points in the direction of the wind (Fig. 9.10). Wind direction is measured from 0 to 360° (degrees).

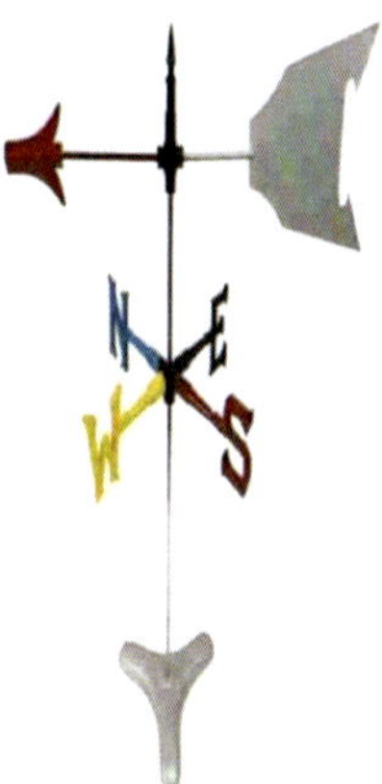

Fig. 9.10: Wind vane

9.4.b. Wind velocity

Wind velocity is generally measured with an anemometer (dial or digital type) and expressed in kilometres per hour (Km/hr), knots (1 knot=1.854 km/hr), or metres per second (m/sec).

9.4.b.1. Cup anemometer

The cup anemometer is a simple type of anemometer. The instrument was invented by Dr. John Thomas Romney Robinson in 1846. In 1926, Canadian John Patterson invented the three-cup anemometer (Fig. 9.11). Later, in 1991, the Australian Derek Weston modified a three-cup anemometer to monitor both wind direction and wind speed.

An anemometer is typically made up of three cups attached to a hub and a photochopper, which produce an electronic signal that is exactly proportional to wind speed. When air passed through the cups in any horizontal direction, it twisted the cups in proportion to the wind speed. As a result, calculating the rotations of the cups over a defined time period produced the average wind speed for a wide range of conditions. The reading is expressed in m/s.

Wind speed is calculated by multiplying the value by the correction factors (Wind speed= reading x default correction factors). Default correction factors are as follows:

Sl.No.	Wind speeds	Correction factors
1	If wind speed is within 5m/s	1.00 m/s
2	Wind speed up to 10m/s	0.98 m/s
3	Wind speed between 10 -15 m/s	0.97 m/s

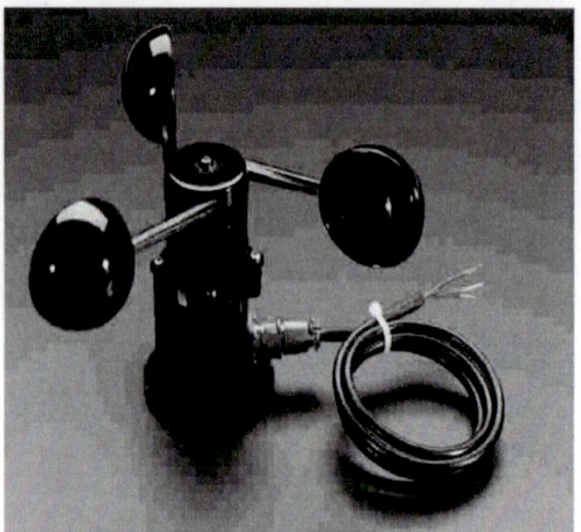

Fig. 9.11: Cup-type anemometer with vertical axis, a photochopper

9.4.b.2. Anemometer (digital type)

A digital anemometer is made up of two parts: an anemometer fan with blades and a screen connected by a wire. This instrument may display the immediate wind velocity in digits (in metres per second, feet per minute, or knots). The 'on', 'off', and 'hold' functions are controlled by an adjustable switch. The wind velocity at a specific point in time is captured using the 'hold' switch.

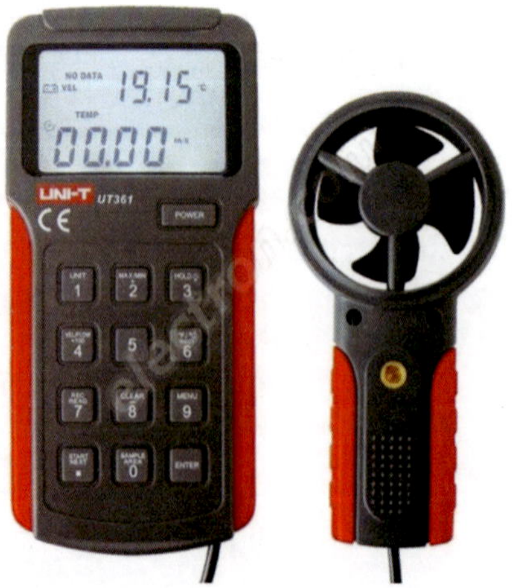

Fig. 9.12: Anemometer (digital type)

9.5. Measurement of Rainfall

Monthly rainfall data can be used to prepare a climatograph for a certain location and time. A climatograph provides precise information about temperature and rainfall in a specific area over the course of a year, allowing better planning for livestock, bird housing, and feeding management in that area. To measure rainfall, rain gauges, snow gauges, and other types of rain gauges are often employed.

9.5.a. Rain gauge

Rain gauges are divided into two types: recording and non-recording. The ordinary or cylindrical rain gauge is consisted of three parts: (a) the collection, (b) the funnel, and (c) the bottle, as shown in Fig 9.12. The diameter of the funnel's rim is 20 cm. The raindrops are collected through the funnel and are accumulated in the bottle. A graduated cylinder is used to measure the collected rain in the bottle. The volume of rainfall is expressed in millimetres or centimetres.

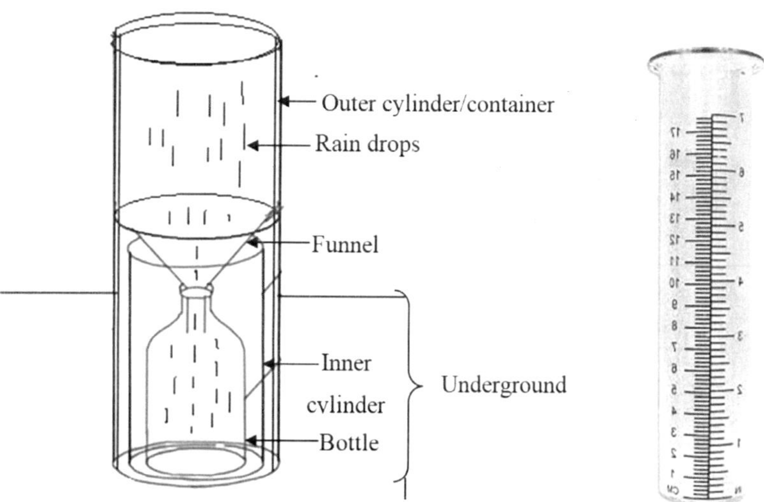

Fig. 9.13: Illustration of different parts of the rain gauge with a graduated measuring cylinder.

In general, the rainwater in the bottle should be measured at 8.30 a.m. every day. It must be measured three or four times each day during heavy rains, after the initial measurement at 8.30 a.m. The rainfall for the day is then calculated by adding all of the measured rainfall over the previous 24 hours.

9.6. Recording of Health or Physiological Parameters

The physiological or health parameters such as body temperature, pulse rate, heart rate, and respiration rate, indicate the animal's physiological state. The physiological parameters' reference values varied according to the age, breed, sex, enthusiasm, environmental stress, and health state of animals.

Animals' respiratory, circulatory, endocrine, neurological, and excretory systems undergo a number of alterations in hot temperatures to maintain homeostasis. These variations can be evaluated by examining physiological parameters. This is why physiological parameters are used to assess animal adaptability. The procedure for recording pulse rate is mentioned in Chapter 2.

9.6.a. Rectal Temperature

In domestic animals, the rectal temperature is used as a proxy for the core body temperature. Rectal temperature is employed in both thermoregulation and diagnostic procedures. Traditionally, animals' rectal temperatures are measured with a clinical mercury thermometer or a digital thermometer.

Materials required

- Clinical thermometer, cotton, liquid paraffin, or glycerin or soap.

Procedure

- Shake the thermometer before recording the temperature to bring it to the beginning of the mercury column.
- Insert the bulb of the thermometer into the rectum, and then tilt it to one side so that the bulb of the thermometer touches the mucous membrane of the rectum. When measuring the rectal temperature of a puppy or kitten, lubricate the thermometer bulb with liquid paraffin, glycerin, soap, or water.
- Keep the thermometer in this position for one minute, and then, take it out, wipe the faces with cotton, and read the temperature directly from the mercury column.

Table 9.3: Reference value for body temperature in domestic animals:

S.No	Animals	Body temperature(°F)
1.	Horse	100.5
2.	Cattle	101.5
3.	Buffalo	101.2
4.	Sheep and Goat	102.5
5.	Pig	102.0
6.	Dog	102.5
7.	Cat	102.0
8.	Bird	105.0-106.0

9.6.b. Respiration Rate

The rate and frequency of respiration differ amongst species. In animals, the following methods can be used to record respiration rate:

I. Paper method

- Count the animal's respiratory rate by placing a paper strip near its nostrils. During inspiration, the paper will move towards the nostrils and away during expiration.
- Count how many times the paper is pushed per minute.

II. Abdominal method or Flank method

- Count the rise and fall of the animal's abdominal flank when standing (distinguish it from the rise and fall of the left abdominal flank during ruminal contraction).
- Count how many times the flank rises per minute.

III. Auscultation method

- Place a stethoscope over the animals' chests.
- Take notes on the breathing sounds you make during inspiration and expiration.
- Count the number of seconds per minute.

Table 9.4: Reference intervals for respiration rate in domestic animals:

S.No	Animals	Respiration rate/ minute
1.	Horse	8-10
2.	Cattle	15-22
3.	Buffalo	15-22
4.	Sheep and Goat	12-20
5.	Pig	10-20
6.	Dog	10-30
7.	Cat	20-30
8.	Bird	15-30

Note: The first observable response of domestic animals to heat stress is respiration rate, which oscillates with the thermal environment.

9.6.c. Heart Rate

Heart rate can be recorded by feeling the pulse, listening to heart sounds, using an electrocardiogram, and telemeter. Listening to heart sounds using a stethoscope is the simplest method of counting the heart rate of domestic animals.

Materials required

- Stethoscope, service crate, animal, etc.

Procedure

- Gently restrain the animal in a quiet room or service crate in case of a large animal and a standing position is preferred.
- Place the chest piece of the stethoscope over the heart and the earpieces into the ear of the observer. The location of the heart in animals varies from species to species.
- Count the number of heartbeats for at least 30 seconds or one minute.

Note: Apart from the health indicator, the shift in heart rate is thought to be related to an adaptation process of the animals to their environment.

9.7. Terminology

- **Absolute humidity (Vapor density):** It refers to a measure of the actual amount of water vapor (moisture) in the air, regardless of the air's temperature.
- **Acclimation:** It refers to certain physiological changes that result from prolonged exposure to a single component of the environment. For

example, acclimation to heat is accompanied by an increase in blood volume.

- **Acclimatization:** It refers to the long-term adaptive physiological adjustments that result in increased tolerance to continuous or repeated exposure to complex climatic stressors. For example, acclimatization to higher altitudes requires acclimatization to both *hypoxia* and *high altitude*.
- **Adaptation**: It refers to the capacity and process of adjustment of an animal to itself, to other living materials, and to the external physical environment. For example, long-haired coats in cold-adapted species and thin coats in heat-adapted species.
- **Adaptation (Biology):** It refers to the morphological, anatomical, physiological, biochemical and behavioural characteristics of the animals, which promote welfare and favor survival in a specific environment.
- **Adaptation (Genetic):** It refers to the heritable animal characteristics which favor survival of a population in a particular environment. This may include evolutionary changes over many generations that acquire specific genetic properties.
- **Adaptation (Physiological):** It refers to the capacity and process of adjustment of the animal to itself to other living material, and its external physical environment.
- **Altitude:** It is the height above the mean sea level in meters or in reference to the standard surface pressure (760 mm of Hg).
- **Bioclimatology:** The branch of climatology that deals with the interrelations between climate, animals, plants, and soils.
- **Climate:** It is the long-term (~some 30 years) average conditions of meteorological variables such as air temperature, humidity, wind velocity, barometric pressure, and solar radiation in a given region.
- **Climatology:** The science that deals with the study of climate.
- **Climatography:** It refers to the quantitative description of the climate which shows the characteristic values of climatic elements for a particular area.
- **External environment:** It is a combination of climatic conditions like solar radiation, air pressure, humidity, interaction with fellow animals, and the temperature under which the animal lives.

- **Internal environment:** It refers to the maintenance of homeostasis of extracellular fluid within the animal body in extreme climatic as well as diseased conditions.
- **Homeostasis:** It is a reaction of the animals to any non-specific environment that involves the pituitary, thyroid, and adrenal glands and tries to place the body in a physiological state.
- **Homeotherms/ Thermal regulator/ Warm blooded/ Endotermia:** Are those animals that maintain a constant body, temperature despite changes in the environmental temperature. For example, large mammals, humans, etc.
- **Humidity:** It is a measure of the vapor content of the air.
- **Macroclimate:** The climate of a large area of the open atmosphere as distinguished from that of a small area.
- **Microclimate:** The climatic condition directly is surrounding the animal.
- **Poikilothermism:** It is a state of changing body temperature with changed environmental temperature. For example, reptiles and amphibians.
- **Precipitation:** It is the form of water particles, liquid, or solid that falls from the atmosphere and reach the ground. It includes rain, snow palates, show grains, ice crystals, etc.
- **Psychromatry:** It is the study of the determination of amount of moisture in the air by the use of a psychrometer or charts.
- **Psychromatric charts:** It is a graph for obtaining relative humidity, absolute humidity, and dew point from dry and wet bulb thermometer readings.
- **Relative humidity:** A ratio of actual vapor pressure of air to the saturated vapor pressure.
- **Weather:** A short-term day-to-day fluctuation of meteorological variables. For example, air temperature, humidity, wind velocity, solar radiation etc.

10

Animal Behaviour

10.0. Introduction

Animal behaviour is the study of how animals interact with one another, other living things, and their environment. Animals display a variety of behaviours in response to both external stimulus and their own pathophysiological state. Almost all domestic animals express a variety of behavioural responses throughout their lifespan, like feeding, sexual behaviours, etc. But every species responds to the same stimuli in a different way. This is why; the study of animal behaviour helps in efficient breeding, feeding, and reproductive management. It also serves as a reliable indicator of overall health and well-being.

10.1. Reproductive Behaviour

Reproductive behaviours are the manifestation of the organism's own reproduction physiology, a system whose foundation is set many months or years before. These include patterns of behaviour related to courting, copulation, birth, maternal care, including newborn suckling attempts, etc. Every species has displayed sexual behaviour. Within species, males and females have different sexual behaviours.

10.2. Male Sexual Behaviour

Male sexual behaviour is innate in nature and it reflects their reproductive efficiency. It is a very complex phenomenon and is determined by the interaction of the organism's internal (hormone and neurological) and external environments. Testosterone, a testicular steroid hormone, is essential for the development and maintenance of normal male sexual behaviour. Genetics, age, experience, nutrition, social environment, temperament, handling, housing, pathologies, or traumatic reasons influence male sexual behaviour.

Male sexual behaviour includes sniffing, licking the female, Flehmen reaction, nuzzling-rubbing the female body surface with the nose, mating or copulation behaviour, etc. Mating or copulation behaviour evolves in sequential steps as follows:

- Sexual arousal or desire (libido)
- Courtship (sexual display) or foreplay
- Penile erection
- Penile protrusion
- Mounting
- Penile intromission
- Orgasm and ejaculation
- Dismounting and refractoriness

One of the most important male sexual activities is the deposition of a sufficient number of viable spermatozoa in the female reproductive tract during estrous or heat. In order to successfully impregnate female animals, the male animal must produce an adequate number of viable spermatozoa as well as have sex desire and mating abilities, especially in natural breeding.

The essential features for the deposition of semen in the female reproductive tract, such as intromission, pelvic thrust, and ejaculation characteristics are almost the same in all males. The length of courtship and intermission in animals varies from species to species. The interval for the bull, ram, and buck is quick, while the stallion takes roughly 40 seconds. Boar requires a longer interval (5-20 minutes). Understanding male sexual behaviour is therefore crucial for effective domestic animal reproductive management.

Table 10.1: Specific male courtship or sexual display in different species:

Animals	Mode of communication	Expression of behaviour
All domestic animal except boar	Chemical communication (through both olfactory and gustatory pathway).	Flehmen reaction. A behaviour in which male animal stand rigidly with their upper lips curled upward after sniffing the female genitalia and urine, to facilitate the transfer of scents and pheromones into the vomeronasal organ above the roof of the mouth via a duct.
Stallion	Tactile communication	Nudging.
Ram, buck andbull	Tactile communication	Nuzzling of the perineal region.
Boar	Tactile communication	Nudging.
Stallion	Auditory communication	Snouts.
Ram	Auditory communication	Baaing.

Male sexual behaviour can be evaluated using a variety of tests. The most routinely employed tests are sexual aggressiveness, reaction time (interval to first service), serving capacity (number of services per test), sex-drive (degree of sexual interest, including mounts and services, mating ability (ratio of mounts to copulations), exhaustion test (copulation rate over time), libido score test, penile erection score, penile protrusion score, ejaculatory thrust score, etc.

Libido in bulls is a heritable trait. The willingness and eagerness of a bull to attempt, mount, and service a female animal is called libido or sex drive. It is sometimes described as sexual motivation.

Materials required

- Breeding bull, service crate, stopwatch, dummy or estrus cow, etc.

Procedure

- Allow the bulls to watch the mating activity in an adjacent pen for at least 5-10 minutes before testing.
- Then restrain an estrus female cow in a service crate.
- Observe the temperament, sexual and mating behaviour indicating sexual interest (e.g., sniffing genitals, licking, grooming, chin resting, tending, Flehmen reaction, etc), attempt to mount or incomplete mount, complete mount without intromission, and service (including intromission and ejaculation). Subsequently, grade the temperament and libido or sex derive as per the scorecard shown below in Tables 10.2 and 10.3, respectively.
- Record the reaction time with a stopwatch. Reaction time is the time lapse between the exposures of the male animal to the female or dummy until successful ejaculation.
- Grade the erection and protrusion of the penis during seeking and ejaculatory thrust, as described below in Table 10.3.

Table 10.2: Temperament scorecard for bull:

S.No	Description of temperament	Score
1	The bull stands very quietly and offers no resistance, only casual hair twitching.	0
2	The bull is generally quiet, offers token resistance, and has steady movement.	01
3	The bull has slightly excited movements, straining and paddling, and may kick.	02
4	The bull is excited and shows vigorous, abrupt movements, straining, and paddling, it may kick.	03
5	The bull is very disturbed, frightened, has wide movements, and may jump and falldown.	04
6	Unmanageable and dangerous.	05

The libido score method assesses both the libido and mating ability of a male animal. Mating ability is the ratio of mounts to copulations.

Table 10.3: Libido scorecard for bull:

S.No	Description of temperament	Score
1	No sexual interest.	0
2	Sexual interests only once, like sniffing at the perineal region.	1
3	Positive sexual interest in females more than one.	2
4	Active pursuit towards females with persistent sexual interest.	3
5	One mount or mounting attempt, no service.	4
6	Two mounts or mounting attempts, no service.	5
7	More than two mounts or mounting attempts, no service.	6
8	One mount or mounting attempts, no service.	7
9	One service followed by further sexual interest, including mounts or mounting attempts.	8
10	Two services followed by no further sexual interest.	9
11	Two services followed by sexual interest including mounting attempts or further services.	10

Table 10.4: Scorecard for penile erection, protrusion and thrust for bulls:

Sl.No	Penile erection score		Protrusion score		Thrust score	
	Description	Score	Description	Score	Description	Score
1	No erection	0	No protrusion	0	No thrust	0
2	Partial erection	01	Partial protrusion	01	Weak thrust	01
3	Fair erection	02	Fair protrusion	02	Good thrust	02
4	Good erection	03	Normal protrusion	03	Very good thrust	03
5	Very good erection	04	Abnormal protrusion	04	Excellent thrust	04

Abnormal male sexual behaviour

Physiological, environmental, and psychological factors determine the intensity of male sexual activity. The common abnormal sexual behaviours are as follows:

- Homosexuality
- Hypo & hypersexuality
- Inability to copulate
- Impotence to mount
- Intromission failure
- Buller- steer syndrome
- Auto-erotic behaviour

- False ejaculation
- Outside ejaculation

10.3. Female Sexual Behaviour

Female sexual behaviour during estrus includes restlessness, loss of appetite, attempting to mount, bellowing, sniffing-particularly the scrotal region of the male, mating position, allowing the males to mount her during estrus, etc. The expression of female sexual behaviour requires interactions between a variety of hormones and social-environmental variables. Ovarian steroid hormones play a crucial role in the expression of sexual behaviour. Estrogen is important for the manifestation of behaviour signs of estrus (prospective behaviour) in many domestic animals. Progesterone is essential for receptive behaviour. Receptive behaviour permits most female domestic animals to stand rigidly for another animal to mount her during estrus.

External factors like odour and pheromones also influence female sexual behaviour in many domestic animals. Pheromones are diverse groups of chemical messengers that relay communications between individuals of the same species in domestic animals. For example-sow will not exhibit immobile receptive sexual behaviour in the absence of odour of a boar or the lack of a mounting attempt. Boar produced 3α-androstenol and 5α-androstenone which affects female in estrus. These pheromones are released through urine, prenuptial secretions, and saliva.

Androstenol is a testosterone metabolite that regulates the sexual behaviours of female animals and is essential for the expression of male sexual behaviour, such as the courting sound or chants de Coeur in boars. In the case of dogs, vaginal secretions contain pheromones called methyl-p-hydroxy benzoate, which is responsible for the attraction of males during estrus. The ram smell induces an increased frequency of pulsatile discharge of LH in ewes.

Estrus is one of the most crucial female sexual behaviors. The intensity of the libido of a female domestic animal is determined based on estrus behavioural signs. The approach is the same as estrus detection in domestic animals based on behavioural signs, as mentioned in Chapter 7. Grade the intensity of estrus in cows based on the following scorecard as shown below in Table 10.5. The success of conception in female animals is greatly dependent on precise estrus detection and time of AI.

Table 10.5: Scorecard for itensity of estrus in cows

Behavioural symptoms	Intense	Intermediate	Weak
Restlessness	+++	+	-
Bellowing	+++	++	+
Licking other animals	++	++	+
Mounting other animals	+++	++	+
Standing to be mounted (confirmatory)	+++	+++	+++
Jerky movement of the lumbosacral region	++	++	+
Arching and stretching of back	++	++	+
Appetite reduction	+	-	-
Decline in milk production	+	-	-

Abnormal female sexual behaviour

- Silent heat
- Nymphomania
- Post-pubertal anoestrus
- Delayed puberty
- Post coital dramatic behaviour in dog and cats

10.4. Feeding Behaviour

Growth and health are intimately correlated with the feeding behaviour of animals. Animals develop distinct feeding habits at a young age that remain constant throughout their lifespan. Neuroendocrine systems integrate the physiology of feeding behaviour. Additionally, environmental factors like management practices and feed quality have a significant impact on animal feeding behaviour. When animals are hungry, they ingest feed to meet their metabolic needs and maintain homeostasis.

The hypothalamus of the brain regulates feeding behaviour and energy balance. When the gastrointestinal system is dilated by ingested feed, the stretch receptors of the gastric pit transmit a signal to the hypothalamus via the vagal afferent nerves, where the efferent signal originates, to restrict feeding behaviours. The humoral mechanism is more complex than neuronal regulation. Several hormones like glucocorticoid, ghrelin, leptin, gonadotropin-inhibitory hormone, estrogen and several neuropeptides like proopiomelanocortin (POMC), neuropeptide-Y (NPY), agouti-related peptide (AgRP), cocaine- and amphetamine-regulated transcript (CART), orexin, cholecystokinin (CCK) and melanin-concentrating hormone (MCH), regulate the physiology of feeding behaviour in most domestic animals.

Increased levels of circulatory ghrelin stimulates feed intake in dairy cattle. When dietary fat and protein reach the small intestine, CCK is released. Across many domestic species, this peptide increases the release of digestive enzymes while inhibiting voluntary feed intake. Similarly, a decrease in appetite in most domestic animals during heat or estrus is caused by higher estrogen levels.

Diet selection and food intake are examples of feeding behaviours. In domestic animals, feeding behaviour differs from species to species. The typical feeding behaviour of cattle in a pasture grazing system is to spend a considerable amount of the day on feeding (grazing behaviour). Cattle and sheep graze approximately 3 and 3-8 miles per day, respectively, mostly throughout the day. Also, they exhibit unusual ruminant behaviour (rumination). Rumination occurs during rest time, especially at night.

Ad libitum and voluntary feed intake are undoubtedly the most important determinants of animal production and welfare. Changes in feeding behaviour are caused by poor health or pain. This is why studying feeding behaviour is important for understanding the impacts of nutrition on digestive function, performance, health, and welfare. It also holds the prospect of new treatment options for feeding-related diseases.

A variety of parameters such as dry matter intake (kg/day), average intake per visit to the feeder (kg/visit), number of visits to the feeder (visits/day), time spent in the feeder (minutes/day), average time per visit (minutes/visit), feeding rate (g/minutes), time spent in rumination, etc. are used for evaluating feeding behaviour in animals.

Feeding behaviour can be measured through direct observation of animals and non-invasive sensor-based automated systems. Under a pasture-free-range management system, direct observation to measure feeding behaviour is labour-intensive, error-prone, and hardly applicable for continuous observations on numerous animals at the same time. However, non-invasive sensor-based systems allow automatic measurement of animal feeding behaviours.

Procedure

- Select a group of animals that are of the same age and weight (in kg) and keep them in separate stalls where they can move around freely with little physical restraints and they can also observe other animals.
- Record the feeding behaviours.
- Prepare an ethogram, either a pie chart or a bar chart, to classify the behaviour that was observed.
- Interpret the findings.

Indication of feeding behaviour

- Rumination and eating habits are crucial indicators for determining the health status of cattle. Decreased rumination time is seen in associated with the onset of calving estrus, stress, anxiety, and diseases such as mastitis, metritis, subclinical ketosis, lameness, etc.
- A nutritional deficiency (pica) in dogs is indicated by abnormal eating behaviours such as devouring objects such as rocks, wood, plastic, strings, rubber bands, and other non-food items.

References

Akhtar N, Jafarikia M, Sullivan, B S and Julang LI (2018) The Journal of Veterinary Medical Science 80(1):147-151.

Banks EP, Jefferson WN and R Retha (2001) Newbold Environmental Health Perspective, 109(8):821-826.

Barnett A J and Reid R L (1956) The Journal of Agricultural Science 48:315-321.

Chenoweth P J (1981)Theriogenology 16:155-170.

Church DC, Editor: The ruminant animal. Digestive physiology and nutrition, Englewood Cliffs, NJ, 1988, Prentice-Hall.

Erwin C and Elting E C (1926) Journal of Agricultural Research 33(3): 269-279.

Fortina R, Patrucco S G, Barbera S and Tassone S (2022). Methods and Protocols 5:59.

Hearnshaw H and Morris C A (1984) Australian Journal of Agricultural Research 35:723-33.

Hoff HE, Geddes LA and McCrady JD (1965) Connecticut Medicine 13(11):795-800.

Jones ML and Allison RW (2007) Veterinary Clinics of North America: Food Animal Practice, 23:377-402.

Joshi V K and Kharche K G (1992) Livestock Advisor17(2):38-41

Kamboj M and Prakash B S (1993) Tropical Animal Health and Production 25:185-19.

McDonald P, Edwards R A, Greenhalgh J F D and Morgan C A (2012) Animal Nutrition (6th Edition), Pearson India Education Services Pvt. Ltd.

Meg M. Sleeper (2020), DACVIM (cardiology) dvm360, 51 (2).

Mondal M, Rajkhowa C and Prakash BS (2006) Hormones and Behavior 49:626–633

Reece W.O (2005) Dukes' Physiology of domestic animals. 12th Edition (Indian Edn) Panima Publishing Corporation.

Rose MK, Gupta M and Sindhu S (2015). Practical Veterinary Physiology. Kalyani Publishers, Civil lines Ludhiana (Punjab)-141008.

Seth M, Jackson, KV, and Giger, U (2011) American Journal of Veterinary Research72,(2):203-9.

Tripathi M K and Karim S A (2008). The Indian Journal of Small Ruminants 41(1) 48.

Warren AL, Stokol T, Hecker KG and Nydam DV (2013) Comparative Clinical Pathology 22:1235-1240.

William O. Reece, Howard H. Erickson, Jesse P. Goff and Etsuro E. Uemura, Editiors Dukes' Physiology of domestic animals. 13th Edition (Indian Edn), 2005, Panima Publishing Corporation.

Zehner N, Umstätter, C, Niederhauser, J J and Matthias Schick M (2017) Computers and Electronics in Agriculture 136: 31-41.

Index